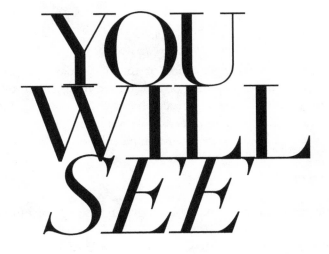

YOU WILL SEE

*walking through uncertainty
and seeing God in it all*

SARAH U. BUCK

Edited by Dara Lynn Rieger

Published by Argyle Fox Publishing | argylefoxpublishing.com

ISBN 978-1-953259-08-0 (Paperback)
ISBN 978-1-953259-09-7 (Ebook)

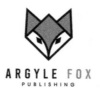

ARGYLE FOX
PUBLISHING

For Forbes

I'm in awe that I get to walk through each day with you.
Thank you for always being my constant.
I love you more than you will ever know.

For Audrey, Warren, and Analise

There are no words to express
the gratitude I feel to be your mom.
Always know that God is
undeniably real and infinitely good.
I love you dearly.

OCEANS

You call me out upon the waters
The great unknown where feet may fail
And there I find You in the mystery
In oceans deep my faith will stand

I will call upon Your Name
And keep my eyes above the waves
When oceans rise
My soul will rest in Your embrace
For I am Yours and You are mine

Your grace abounds in deepest waters
Your sovereign hand will be my guide
Where feet may fail and fear surrounds me
You've never failed and You won't start now

Spirit lead me where my trust is without borders
Let me walk upon the waters
Wherever You would call me
Take me deeper than my feet could ever wander
And my faith will be made stronger
In the presence of my Saviour

I will call upon Your Name
Keep my eyes above the waves
My soul will rest in Your embrace
I am Yours and You are mine[1]

-Hillsong United

CONTENTS

Prologue • 13

YOU WILL SEE

PROLOGUE

LAUNDRY. IT HAD MY number.

I stood at the base of the staircase and stared at the twelve steps in front of me wondering, *How is this going to work? How am I going to get this overflowing basket of clean clothes up all those stairs?*

It was only twelve steps.

I could hear my two small children playing in the next room. Not a care in the world. I smiled at the sweet sound of their voices.

I can't ask them for help. I'm the mom. This is my job! My pride flinched at the thought of asking my little ones to help me.

Steeling my resolve, I slowly lifted the heavy load onto the first step, then turned around to sit down next to it. I took a deep breath and proceeded to inch myself up each step while pulling the basket up with my good hand. Even those incredibly slow movements sent stinging pain throughout my entire body. But, I wasn't about to ask for help.

I've given birth, TWICE. I can get this laundry basket up the stairs.

Or at least I thought I could. But, the basket was too full, and I was too weak. Every time I inched it up, another piece of clean clothing fell out and rolled down the stairs, taunting me as it slid out of reach.

This unbelievably slow system had seemed like a logical way to get this impossible chore done. Instead, it was totally inefficient and more than a little demoralizing. I'm glad no one was there to watch, or heaven forbid, try to "help me."

Why is this so hard?

But, I refused to surrender to the laundry gods or wave a clean, white t-shirt in defeat. Determined, I pulled as hard as I could and, with my last ounce of strength, made it to the top. Too weak to stand after all that effort, I slowly scooted back down the stairs to gather the trail of dropped pairs of underwear and socks.

And that was when the dam broke.

Suddenly, I was overwhelmed by a flood of tears. There was nothing I could do to hold them back. I'm not sure if I was crying because I was in so much pain, or because I couldn't do something as mundane as laundry. Everything just felt hard as I tried desperately to adjust to the changes in my abilities. It felt like my body was betraying me.

After the tears, I found myself in a hazy daydream about my children's favorite cartoon, *Jake and the Neverland Pirates*. I thought about Izzy and her penchant for pixie dust. She could simply toss it in the air to take her pirate friends anywhere they needed to go. (Here's to all the mamas who now have that theme song stuck in their head.) I pondered how great it would be to fling a little pixie dust around and float up those stairs with my perfectly folded clothes sailing alongside. I smiled at the thought of getting to be my own version of the fairy godmother . . . of laundry.

I would wave my arms around, directing blue jeans, t-shirts, pajamas, and perfectly-paired socks to their rightful drawers. But, then I snapped back to reality and looked around at the now unfolded pile in my lap. What had taken me four times longer than normal to fold was now a wasted effort.

This was a new low.

I realized that my life was a lot like that laundry. Just a few months before it had been simple, easy, and routine. But, now it was messy, difficult, and undone.

At this point, I had seen at least fifteen doctors and still had zero answers. Not one of them could figure out what was going on inside my body. I couldn't swallow food. I could barely hold my children.

My hands were unrecognizable, drawing in like claws. One side of my body was much weaker than the other.

I kept thinking, *I'm too busy and too young to be taken out by some no-name "thing."* It was becoming more and more challenging to pretend that everything was fine.

I was weak and ached all over. On top of that, I had run out of patience a good while back. If I'd had a gauge to indicate the energy I had left in me to fight, it was stuck way below "E." I was literally running on fumes . . . and pureed vegetables.

But, in spite of the pain, the uncertainty, and my growing list of symptoms, I could feel God's nearness. His presence was with me in ways that were undeniable. For eighteen months, I'd had no answers, but I still had hope. My body had deteriorated, but my faith was growing. Every day brought new challenges and some really painful realities.

But, God was with me during those deeply dark days. And, were it not for Him, I wouldn't be here to tell you my story.

Meanwhile, the moment we get tired in the waiting, God's Spirit is right alongside helping us along. If we don't know how or what to pray, it doesn't matter. He does our praying in and for us, making prayer out of our wordless sighs, our aching groans. He knows us far better than we know ourselves, knows our pregnant condition, and keeps us present before God. That's why we can be so sure that every detail in our lives of love for God is worked into something good. (Romans 8:26–28 MSG)

Part 1

WALKING THROUGH *MYSTERY*

{ *chapter one* }

LIFE BEFORE

Wake up!
Strengthen what remains and is about to die,
for I have found your deeds unfinished
in the sight of my God.

Revelation 3:2

EIGHTEEN MONTHS BEFORE THE laundry basket moment, my life looked dramatically different. I was at the top of my game, running a successful children and infant photography business in my hometown. At thirty, my energy level was boundless. Sleep was something I did for four to five hours a night because, you know, everyone else was doing it, so why not me? In fact, I ate, slept, worked, and breathed at a pace no normal person would attempt to sustain. I was always in a hurry to get to the next thing. If I wanted to stop and smell the roses, I could do it without actually stopping. I was a woman on a mission.

In early 2011, I was happily married to Forbes (still am!)

and mom to two sweet children. Audrey, my three-year old, was serious, loving, and smart. She was the easiest baby and slept through the night at six weeks. That easiness carried into her toddler years. She was passed around quite a bit as a baby and toddler due to my constantly changing work schedule. There were weeks when work got so crazy that she might have napped in four different places, either with a friend, a babysitter, or at my parents' home. As long as she had a good nap, some art supplies, a book, and some goldfish, that sweet girl was happy as a lark.

On the other hand, my seven-month old baby Warren was—well, I hate to say it—an absolute handful. Colic, a milk allergy, and his mama being his favorite made for some trying times. But for the most part, his cuteness and snuggles made up for all the crying. He had a difficult time sleeping those first seven months, and I tried everything under the sun, from crying it out to making a soothing music playlist to get that kid to sleep. I'm not even kidding about the playlist. Want to know what I named it? "Warren Stop Crying." Ha! For the record, Warren transitioned into an easy toddler and became my carefree kiddo with the sweetest personality, which was very fortunate for what lay ahead for our family.

Even in the midst of colicky babies and long work days, my husband and I always made an effort to spend time with each other. During our dating years, we had a standing date night set for the last Friday of every month. Regardless of what was going on around us, we stuck hard to those dates. Forbes even proposed on one of those special date nights.

As our family grew, date nights weren't as consistent as they once were, but we cherished any time we were able to have to ourselves. Forbes has always been my constant. When life has

20

swayed one way or another, he's been there to ground me. It amazes me that two people from two different cities and two very different childhoods could end up together and become so uniquely intertwined that one can't survive without the other. That's the beauty of marriage. Forbes and I have always had an unspoken confidence in our relationship that goes deeper than words can say. It's funny to me that someone as pridefully independent as I am could learn to be so dependent on someone else.

During this time, my job was my life and I loved every single part of it. Even though most of my shoots were outdoors, the coastal heat never bothered me. I'll admit that the bugs occasionally got on my nerves, but when I had a camera in my hand, the whole world opened up and I saw life differently. I always experienced a unique depth to God's presence whenever I was behind a camera.

This season of life had me running all the time and I didn't let anything slow me down. I was always excited to have new clients and never turned down the chance to take on more business. Providing my clients with exceptional work and climbing that proverbial ladder of success was my main focus, and I let everything else come a close second.

Regardless of how late I pored over client photos, the alarm was still set for 5 a.m. so I could exercise, edit photos, drink a pot of coffee, and then head to the first shoot of the day. And while I worked crazy hours and long days, my husband did the very same thing at his job as an accountant. We were both in the prime time of our lives, building careers and driven to succeed. Looking back now, I can see that even as we did the best we could, we robbed ourselves of a lot of downtime and stayed stressed, even working on holidays.

Life was busy, but in the midst of all that, there were still moments that felt timeless. Nothing compared to coming home sweaty and covered in marsh mud from an outdoor photo shoot and being loudly greeted by happy children as I hosed myself off on the back porch. Audrey, and later Warren, were notorious for flinging the back door open as they raced to greet me, which caused the door to slam against the house, shaking the blinds and making quite the racket. Being welcomed home with sweet, sometimes sticky, hugs from my kiddos was always the best part of my day.

We lived in a mid-century brick house on a corner lot in a cozy neighborhood. The house had been my great aunt's years before and all the memories I had on her back porch from childhood came to life when my kids were outside playing in the backyard. Everything about that back porch reminded me of my aunt and the dedication she had to loving us BIG. It was such a gift to have a home with so many good memories attached to it.

This house also had significance because it was where we brought our babies home. It was where I had my first photography studio and where we would spend the most difficult years of my illness. It became a refuge and a safe retreat for one of the hardest seasons I've ever walked through.

As the years rolled on, I worked my tail off to own the family photography market in our hometown. By the time I got to the top and was in such demand that I had wait lists, I noticed a little tug on my heart. Do you ever get those? Those moments when you realize that everything you've worked so hard to achieve doesn't make you feel the way you thought it would? I made it to where I thought I wanted to be and discovered it could not have been further from what I really wanted.

Don't get me wrong. I *loved* what I did for a living. It was an absolute honor to photograph each newborn baby, family, and big life moment. To this day, I remember many children's birthdays, because I was there when they took their first breaths in the delivery room. Many of the friends I've made since moving back to my hometown after college are my clients. There is something really special about being responsible for documenting the lives of so many children. I get the warm fuzzies thinking about it. I also do that old lady thing when I run into them in a restaurant or Target (my favorite store) and tell them, "I can't believe how big you've gotten! I remember the day you were born!" The thing is though, I *really* do remember the day they were born and how grateful I was that God allowed me the privilege of capturing each of those moments. All this to say, I loved my clients, their children, and the many fun memories we had along the way. In the thirteen years that I ran my business, I can only think of one less-than-great moment during a shoot, which we all laugh about now. To this day, I'm still so grateful my clients didn't make fun of me to my face during their shoot when I fell flat on my tush in the water with my camera held high up in the air!

Despite my love for my job and my gratefulness for the talent God gave me to do it, reaching the level of success I longed for didn't fulfill me in the least. Somewhere along the way, I began to value the talent God had given me more highly than I valued Him. I knew I had to work on getting my priorities in line. Even though I felt God's presence every time I picked up a camera and a tangible closeness to Him when I was working, my heart was desperately needing more of Him.

I'm not sure of the exact moment when that tug on my heart first happened, but I'm pretty sure it was a gradual nudge that slowly became more undeniable over a few months. I was stressed and torn between the balance of children, the rat race of work, the relentless pursuit of success, and maintaining a social presence. During all of it, I never really felt at peace. Sadly, my priorities were in line with the Gospel According to Sarah.

I loved God, thanked Him for the blessings He continued to give me, read my devotions faithfully, and tried to do all the good Christian things. But somewhere along the way with getting married, having children, and trying to be successful, my priorities shifted drastically. Yes, we attended church regularly, and yes, I did have a relationship with Jesus. But I'm kidding myself and you if I claim God was my first priority. He had been at other times in my life, especially in high school and the beginning of college, but as my personal independence grew, my dependence on God began to fade. That shift can happen so easily, often without our being aware of it.

And so, in the midst of all the busyness and the striving for success that had me completely distracted, God was reaching out to me, calling me to Himself. I could feel Him gently tugging at my heart, so I started spending more time with Him. Soon after, one of my closest friends invited me to a women's retreat at her church. The camaraderie was a gift, as was the feeling that I was being fed spiritually in a way I'd never been before. During that weekend, as I listened to speakers and was inspired to live more fully, I had no idea that within a few short hours my life would change forever.

God's timing is perfect, friends. He doesn't waste one moment, one experience, or one hurt. During this time, as God was showing me that things had to change, I got one of those phone calls that no one ever wants to get. A friend of mine was going through a devastatingly hard time and when people get desperate, they do desperate things. In His providence, God chose me to walk with my friend through a difficult season. And in the midst of that experience, God showed me how far I had moved away from Him over the ten years after college. As He graciously walked with my friend and I on a journey that resulted in my friend's healing, He also gave me the wake-up call I needed.

And just like that, ten years of mediocre faith was exposed and God made it clear that was not what He wanted for me. That desperate phone call from my friend was the turning point that began to lead where God wanted to take me. And while I wish my friend never had to suffer through that experience, I'm grateful that God used it to wake me up to Himself in order to prepare me for what was to come.

{ *chapter two* }

IS SOMETHING WRONG?

If any of you lacks wisdom, you should ask God,
who gives generously to all without finding fault,
and it will be given to you.

James 1:5

RUNNING IS ONE OF my great loves. But as much as
I love to run, I had never run a half-marathon. So in the fall of
2011, my best bud Elizabeth (who had several half-marathons
under her belt) talked me into signing up for my first one. We
trained and trained, talked and trained, and ate and trained, all
quite beautifully. We did everything by the book and stuck to a
strict exercise and nutrition regimen to set ourselves up for a
successful run.

As race day got closer, I was ready to put my hard work
and training to the test. The day finally arrived and it was cold.
Very cold. Elizabeth and I put on layers of clothes that we
could peel off as the miles flew by. I can proudly say that we
finished our race in two hours and five minutes! Forbes and the

kids were waiting for me at the finish line, and I have the most embarrassing photo of me running across it with my arms in the air. That picture captured every bit of the joy I felt! We had worked *so* hard.

The excitement overwhelmed me, and I could barely stand up afterwards! No, literally, I collapsed almost immediately after the race and was sick for the rest of the day. Come to find out, I hadn't prepared as well as I thought I had. I was so dehydrated that it took a good twenty-four hours to fully recover. But regardless of how I felt physically, my heart was happy to have finally accomplished something I wasn't sure I could do. Kudos to my training buddy and also to my family who thought I was insane for doing a half marathon, but still graciously helped me out in every way possible to get my miles in.

Several weeks after the run, I was still feeling pretty worn out. I called Elizabeth one morning while packing orders and sipping coffee on the floor of my studio. We caught up for a bit and then she yawned loudly. I laughed and said, "Wow, that was a loud one." She laughed, too, and said, "Gosh, I'm just so worn out. I feel like a Mack truck hit me." I would never have confessed that I was feeling worn out, but since she had shared, I quickly responded, "Me too!" It was somewhat of a relief to know she felt the same way, because it was unfamiliar to me to feel anything other than 100 percent. Because we seemed to be feeling the same tiredness, it never crossed my mind that something could actually be wrong with me. Obviously, it was just a phase that would eventually pass.

Not long after that conversation, it was revealed that Elizabeth's "Mack truck" was, in fact, her now spunky daughter. I knew that was definitely not the reason for my extra fatigue.

In January 2012, after wrapping up the busy Christmas

season of work, I started feeling something I'd never felt before. The worn-out feeling had turned into utter exhaustion.

At this point, our daughter, Audrey, was four and a half and our son, Warren, was eighteen months old. Warren had finally come through that mind-numbing season of crying/no sleeping and was transitioning into being a really enjoyable baby. So I couldn't even blame my lack of energy on him.

At first, the extreme tiredness was just a nuisance. Anyone who knew me would never use the word *tired* to describe me. My pseudo-spiritual gift seemed to be operating joyfully on very little sleep. At first, I chalked up my lethargy to the combo of work and Christmas. But every day, no matter what I did, the fatigue kept getting worse. Most days I woke up feeling like I just couldn't make it out of the bed. After finally managing that, an hour later I would have a terrible sick feeling that lasted all day. It was a lot like having the flu, just without the fever and chills.

Those closest to me would acknowledge that I suffer from an unreal amount of stubbornness, which stems from my overwhelming struggle with prideful self-sufficiency. I *could not* for the life of me accept that I, the health nut (or so I thought), the runner who could run circles around all my friends, actually had a health problem I could not fix. But six weeks into feeling sick and tired, barely able to make it to 8 o'clock at night, I finally decided to see my doctor. It took me those same six weeks to confess to Forbes that I wasn't feeling myself. He was working late hours because it was tax season, and I'm sure he thought it was weird that I was asleep when he got home. But he never said anything. One morning, I nonchalantly mentioned that I was feeling a little low and was going to make an appointment with my doctor.

Up until this point, other than some gastrointestinal issues, I was a healthy girl! I didn't even have an internal medicine doctor, so I went to my OB/GYN. I'm so thankful this is where I started because I'd been consistently going to this practice for five years. The nurse practitioner, Martha, had seen me through one very easy pregnancy and one very hard. She had also seen me bounce back from both, and she and my doctor had been incredibly supportive of my business by connecting me with our local hospital to do birth photography. Needless to say, these folks knew me well.

I'll never forget sitting on the edge of the exam table, looking into Martha's eyes and saying, "I think I must be anemic or something because I have never been this tired or felt this sick in my life." Then I took a deep breath and before I knew it, the flood gates opened.

I'm normally not much of a crier or even a very emotional person, but it was as if I'd been holding it all in until this moment and just couldn't control myself. I told the doctor and nurse practitioner how awful I felt, that I'd been trying to carry on like everything was okay. But everything was not okay.

Because I had a relationship with this practice and they knew I was an early riser and avid runner, they thought further investigation was warranted. Looking back now, I can see that this is the first of many moments when God revealed Himself through people He placed in my life. Martha's compassion motivated me to take the next step in pursuing answers. Over the span of my health journey, she consistently offered encouragement and frequent pep talks. I love how God strategically places people in our lives at certain times to breathe life into us. It's such a good reminder that we aren't meant to do life alone.

IS SOMETHING WRONG?

Following my OB/GYN's orders, I went to the first of many appointments with various internal medicine doctors. At this point, I decided to confess to my mom that I wasn't feeling quite like myself. Motherly intuition is always spot on, and it seemed she'd been waiting for this confession, because she already knew. It was a relief that she knew, but I was hesitant to describe exactly how I felt because I didn't want her to worry.

Over the next couple weeks, between the time I saw the first internal medicine doctor and returned for my blood work results, I lost seven pounds. The doctor told me all my blood work was completely normal and that if the weight loss kept up, I should probably see a gastroenterologist. I remember walking out and saying under my breath, "Hey, thanks for nothing, lady!"

A few weeks later, the fatigue got better, but I was still losing weight. You want to know what the funny part was? People started telling me how great I looked! I felt horrible, but because I was now quite thin, I was looking "great." This is a problem, people! When a healthy person with a healthy weight and lifestyle starts looking emaciated, don't compliment them. Make sure they are okay! Or at least offer them a burger!

As the months went on, my fatigue came and went, but overall got better. However, new symptoms began creeping up. The most annoying of these new symptoms was a diminished memory, which kept me from coming up with the right words in conversation. It took me two months to realize that I had forgotten my niece's birthday and a few other pretty important life events. Birthdays are my jam, so the fact that I totally forgot my sweet niece turning eight was mortifying to me. Then, there were phone calls with clients I'd worked with for years, clients I was in the room with when their kids were born, and their kids' names were completely erased from my mind. Talk about embarrassing. At this point, I was still hiding the fact that anything was wrong with me, so I couldn't even come up with a good excuse for my weird behavior.

Another symptom was that sounds were suddenly bothering me. It felt like every noise was magnified to an unbearable volume that I couldn't turn down, sending chills down my spine. My worried mom was checking in with me daily and I knew she was checking in for my dad too. Some days I took the opportunity to be honest and other days I would go into complete shut-down mode. It felt like if I just didn't talk about it, it wasn't real. As the symptoms became more alarming, there was the question of how to present those to my mom without worrying her while still being honest. There was an art to it, and some days I did better than others.

Then, I started experiencing pain. Real pain. My arms started hurting all the time. As the months went on, the pain in my arms kept me up at night. It was like a brutal combo of bone and nerve pain. Photo shoots became more difficult, but I kept plugging along. The hardest thing about the arm pain was lifting Warren into his crib. I'm not sure why this particular motion was so difficult, but it was. I came up with a method where I turned him onto his stomach, scooped him up, and then shimmied him down my arms into the crib. Thank goodness he was an easier baby at this point and didn't push back at my new and unusual ways of holding him.

Clearly my body was trying to tell me something was wrong. I was desperate for a solution and thought maybe it would help to fuel my body with healthy nutrients. I started taking all kinds of vitamins trying to feel better. But it felt like the vitamins were getting stuck in my throat, which wasn't a feeling I'd ever experienced before. I wasn't sure if it was just a sensation or an actual physiological issue. I went to see our local ENT who thought it could be a symptom of reflux, so I took his suggestions and the medication he prescribed and kept on trucking.

While experiencing all these unusual symptoms, I was totally unable to find a solution to them on my own. That uncomfortable feeling of the vitamins getting stuck in my throat is a lot like the uncomfortable situation I was in. I had quickly become stuck in a predicament I couldn't fix by myself.

Being stuck is not a fun place to be, and there are so many ways we can get stuck. Stuck in broken relationships, stuck putting too much effort in the wrong direction, stuck on misconstrued ideas about what we think is happening to us or what we believe people think of us. You get the idea. When we get to a place in life where we don't know how to move forward anymore, much like those vitamins getting stuck in my throat, we just stop. Life keeps moving around us, but we don't know how to operate anymore, so we just do what we have to do in order to get by. But in that place, there's no going forward, no real growth or change of any kind. In those moments, we can grow numb and the desire to move ahead vanishes.

Something outside of ourselves has to make it possible for us to become *unstuck*. Proverbs 28:13 says that "whoever conceals their sins does not prosper, but whoever confesses and renounces them finds mercy." Being honest about our overwhelming need for God is the first step to getting unstuck. You can't hide anything from God, so you might as well come clean and confess to the One who knows all about what's going on. Every time I've found myself stuck, I'm usually pretty aware of how I got there. When I try doing it myself, I never seem to get out of whatever pit I'm in. I stubbornly try to skip the part where I confess what I've been up to, because that makes it all too real. But when I do that and try to fix things myself, I miss out on seeing God do what He does best. He rescues people like me who are stuck in a situation or a feeling they can't get out of by themselves.

So that's where I was. Stuck in a place I was unequipped and powerless to navigate out of on my own.

I'm not sure why surrendering is so hard to do. The simplicity of surrendering is that by giving God complete control, we receive so much freedom.

God has used all sorts of avenues to teach me this lesson of surrender. One of those has been parenthood. Being a parent is a great way to find out that we're all basically the same stubborn, strong-willed children we once were, just a little taller and with a few more responsibilities. These days, God regularly teaches me about my own sin nature and my "do-it-myself" tendencies while parenting my kiddos.

Not long ago, I heard my toddler barreling down the hall toward my bathroom yelling, "This is not working! This is not working!" Her tone and volume made me stop what I was doing and wait for her to come around the corner, anxious to see what the problem was. In she walked with her sweater over her head, unsuccessfully trying to squeeze her head through the arm hole, while her arm stuck awkwardly out of the neck hole. If I'm being honest, it was hysterical. She is the most independent child I've ever met, so there was some serious toddler anger involved with her not being able to dress herself that morning. I smiled down at her as she kept bellowing, "It's not working!" Finally, she stopped, let her arms drop in defeat, and looked up at me. When her eyes met mine, she and I laughed together because it was such a funny predicament. But it wasn't until she looked up at me and realized the ridiculousness of her situation that she acknowledged she needed help and couldn't do it on her own.

That's us every single day. We get up ready for the day ahead, prepared for and capable of doing our daily tasks. We take on life in our own strength, because we think we know how. Then there's an inevitable road block and we get stuck, waving our arms and shouting helplessly, "This is not working!"

What if the moment we hit that road block, we looked up and asked for help right then? Sometimes we wallow for months, even years, trying to do things on our own before we realize that we need to literally let Jesus take that proverbial wheel.

I know I would get a lot less stuck in life if I lived everyday with the gospel of Jesus in the forefront of my mind and on the tip of my tongue. What a difference it would make if I woke up every morning acknowledging that I can't get myself unstuck, and that God, in His mercy, sent Jesus to do that for me!

The health journey that was ramping up was about to take me into the wilds of God's providence and His love. I had no idea all the ways He was about to free my heart from its determination to do it myself. Rescue was coming. I just didn't know the lengths it would take or the many mountains and valleys I would have to go through to get there. What I did know was that God would be with me every step of the way.

{ *chapter three* }

TRYING NEW THINGS

I love you, Lord, my strength.
The Lord is my rock, my fortress and my deliverer;
my God is my rock, in whom I take refuge,
my shield and the horn of my salvation, my stronghold.

Psalm 18:1–2

SPRING ARRIVED WITH COLORFUL blooms and warmer weather and, for me, the continued search for answers. By now, I was already on my second internist and, thankfully, he showed a little more compassion than the first. He seemed genuinely concerned over my symptoms. I was losing weight, felt terrible, had extreme shortness of breath, and was experiencing swallowing issues, nausea, and more. He ordered chest CTs, blood work, and stress tests, all of which came back normal.

After digging into things as far as he thought he could, he decided I was likely experiencing anxiety. He offered to write me a prescription for anxiety medicine. And so it went. I felt the deep disappointment of another dead end. While I appreciated his suggestions, I knew myself well enough to know this wasn't anxiety. I also knew something was wrong, and I desperately wanted answers.

Truly, I had many friends get involved at this point to help. Well, the ones who knew what I was dealing with. Remember, at this point I was still a super prideful person, so I only allowed my closest friends and those who could help me know what was really going on. I'm still surprised by how prideful I can be.

By April, every internal organ I owned was killing me. Honestly, I had no idea where all these organs were located until they each started to ache. Kidney pain became an obvious issue to investigate, so off to a nephrologist I went. A friend of our family contacted a brilliant local nephrologist and he took a stab (literally, like fifty tubes of blood) at getting to the bottom of this mystery. By now, I was looking pretty rough and my coloring was off, so it wasn't hard to convince any doctor that I wasn't feeling well.

The results came back and *everything was normal.* NORMAL! But *nothing* about my life was normal. It's kind of funny that I heard that word more during those abnormal months than at any time in my whole life. The irony is that, for as long as I could remember, I had always been striving for normalcy.

Coming from a divorced family, the moment my parents' marriage was broken, normal completely went out of the window. I did recover some normalcy when my mom remarried and my stepdad adopted me in high school. Then, all of us under one roof shared the same last name. For some reason, sharing a name was really important to me. For me, there was beauty and order embedded in that one small detail. From that moment on, I determined to pursue whatever I thought *normal* was supposed to look like. And now, years later, here I was, being told by these diagnostic results that everything was normal when I knew that everything was very clearly the complete opposite.

Every day, regular things became a little bit harder and I learned the art of "fake it 'til you make it." Normal, everyday gatherings now required every ounce of energy I had. Every birthday party my kids were invited to took enormous effort. You'd think I would have just politely declined to attend, but I wanted things to stay as normal as they could for Audrey and Warren. Invitations would arrive in the mail and I would sigh as I stuck them on the fridge. Before every event, I would psych myself up before getting out of the car. I was thankful for God's strength to sustain me and, to tell the truth, I was also really thankful for make-up!

I got so good at faking it that when friends found out I wasn't doing well, they were shocked. I'd seemed fine when they last saw me. I fought so hard to be perceived as "fine" for a long time. It took more effort and emotional energy than I'd like to admit. Simple things like parties or receptions where I'd have to make small talk or stand around holding a plate of food or laugh at jokes left me drained and in pain for days.

As things worsened, I decided that maybe I should take matters into my own hands, so I found a book about clean eating and detoxing. It's the only book I've ever read in one day. At this point, I was nothing if not determined. On the day after my birthday I cut out all my favorite foods and drinks, which included my beloved coffee. Meanwhile, I was still running my photography business full time, despite everything going on. I literally felt sicker as each day went by. It was like a combo of the feeling you have after recovering from a terrible stomach bug and the flu simultaneously. Every move took enormous effort. My cognitive behavior was also off, and I was forgetting everything.

One particular morning, soon after I'd quit coffee, I showed up to my first photoshoot with zero caffeine in my system. Big mistake. Adding insult to injury, the photoshoot was with a new client and her two beautiful girls. The entire time, I felt like I was in a tunnel. Whenever I would stand or sit, which happens often during photoshoots, I blacked out. I started worrying that my client noticed my unusual behavior, so I decided to throw myself under the bus and acknowledge that I was a little out of it. I explained how I had decided to give up coffee recently and it was affecting me more than I expected. I admitted to her, and maybe to myself, that I had no idea how much caffeine had helped me live my life. She smiled sweetly and gave me a look that I translated to, *Why the heck would you ever give up coffee, lady?* And on we went with the photoshoot.

The day went on and proverbial dark clouds kept descending as things went from bad to worse. I decided to relieve the sitter early and drop by the grocery store for more clean-eating supplies with small kids in tow. I was on the bread aisle in the middle of the store when it all hit me like a truck running into a concrete wall. My vision started to flicker in and out and I thought, *Hmmmm, maybe I can't actually do this. Am I, in fact, insane?*

I feebly pulled out my phone and called my mom who happened to be close by. I told her I was in the middle of Publix, that I literally could not function, and could she, please, come help me? My mom knows me well and was obviously concerned about my recent decline. The fact that I was finally asking for help after refusing it for so long created a sense of urgency for her.

I think my body was in a sort of deprivation shock and the caffeine drip I'd been on had literally been keeping me upright. Mom swooped in like a superhero, grabbing the buggy and my two bundles of joy. She informed me lightly that I was having a migraine as she checked me out at the register. After she drove us home, I don't remember what else happened that day other than dropping into bed. (For those who suffer from migraines, which includes my mom and sister, I genuinely feel for you. I can't think of anything more miserable.) Despite this experience, I stuck with the no-caffeine thing and the detox diet for a while, both which actually gave me some relief for a bit. Although, I use the word *some* here rather loosely.

(A side note seems appropriate to give you a better idea of how deep my need for coffee goes and how desperate I was to get better. Every morning after giving up coffee, I would brew Forbes his coffee and then stand at the stove, whisking together warmed almond milk and raw cacao powder in a pot. As I poured that concoction into a mug, I'd pretend with every sip that it was my beloved coffee. This sad little scenario went on for months, probably five or so. I was determined to do anything to feel better even if it meant drinking a really terrible substitute for coffee.)

Something You Could See

That spring, I saw a few doctors who tested me for random things like Lyme disease, MS, and other possibilities that seemed consistent with my symptoms. One morning in May, I woke up and moved to get out of bed, but my body wasn't moving right. Weird new pains and feelings were the norm these days and I never knew how I would wake up or what I would feel like. I would often wonder as my head hit the pillow at night, *What's tomorrow going to bring?* Some days I would wake up with Bell's Palsy, some days it was stabbing pain in different parts of my body, and some days I had nausea so intense I could barely open my mouth.

But this particular day, I went to take a step forward and my left leg had a delay. This outward physical symptom was the first sign anyone could actually see with their own eyes. It validated that something was, in fact, going on with me! It was like a gift *and* a curse, and I celebrated and grieved simultaneously. For one thing, it was noticeable and now everyone could visibly tell something was clearly wrong. It was embarrassing, but it was also helpful because it was new information. This was how I had started looking at every new symptom, like a detective searching for clues. Each symptom represented a piece to the overall puzzle.

All along I knew Forbes believed everything I said about how I felt and what I was experiencing. I was never much of a complainer, so when I was honest about a new symptom, he always validated me. Even though he understood me, there was a lot of stuff that I didn't vocalize to him. Obviously, this new leg-dragging thing really disturbed him. He was already holding in all of his sadness and frustration about my declining health. Adding my new dramatic neurological symptoms only compounded his fears. Little did we know, it would get worse before it got better.

By this point, I was pretty good at putting on a brave face. Having to be casual about a dragging leg, however, would take some serious skill. Yet again, I doggedly carried on, unwilling to slow my business down or let anything hinder my work. I'll never forget the first time someone asked if I was okay.

I was on a shoot in a downtown park with one of my favorite families. We were searching for some shade, when the husband turned to me and asked, "Are you okay?" Instantly, my face got hot as I inexplicably felt fury and then shame wash over me. What could I say? I thought I was doing such a good job overcompensating for my dragging leg, but apparently, I thought wrong. As embarrassed as I was, I knew he was asking out of genuine concern. "Yeah," I replied, "I have some weird stuff going on and my doctors are trying to figure it out."

This man was also a doctor, so I knew he was at least a little curious about my symptoms. Though he didn't ask questions, he voiced his concern, telling me to let him know if we needed anything. That was one of the first times I had to confess to a client that I wasn't doing well. Along the way, so many of my clients had become my friends. Through this first confession God showed me, *See, that wasn't so terrible, was it?* This particular family stayed connected with us and checked in on me over the next few years. Even when I couldn't do photo shoots, I would get an occasional text from them asking how I was doing.

Maybe you're wondering why it was so hard for me to admit that something was wrong. Growing up, strength wasn't something I worked toward. It was something I felt was required of me. It was something I demanded of myself. But somewhere along the way, I misunderstood strength and weakness. I viewed weakness as failure and strength as control.

As I got back into the car after this particular shoot, God reminded me of Paul's words in 2 Corinthians 12:9: "My grace is sufficient for you, for *my power is made perfect in weakness.*" In that moment, a familiar verse I'd heard my whole life became rich with meaning for me. It gave me confidence to move forward as well as a deep desire to shed more of my "self" so that I could lean further into the strength of the One who was carrying me through this journey.

In Ephesians, the Apostle Paul encourages believers to "be strong in the Lord and in the strength of his might" (Ephesians 6:10 ESV). I love what J.D. Greear, well-known pastor and theologian, has to say about this in his study on Ephesians:

> How strong you are is irrelevant. In fact, your strengths can become a liability in spiritual warfare because those places where you feel strong are the places you're most likely to forget your need to depend on God. In fact, if you feel weak and unqualified to engage in the spiritual realm, that's actually a good thing, because you're more likely to lean on God's power than someone who feels strong. If dependence [on the Lord] is the objective, then weakness becomes an advantage. Beware your strengths, not your weaknesses because your strengths are those places where you're most likely to forget God.[2]

Weakness is an advantage? This was a life-changing shift in perspective for me. Because of my debilitating symptoms, I was beginning to experience something I had never imagined—the freedom to stop trying so hard.

I was literally knee-deep in weakness at this point. Once we saw that my leg dragging wasn't going away, I knew my next stop was the neurologist. Over the next year, I actually saw four of them. The first was by far the most caring, most knowledgeable, and most curious about my condition. He performed so many tests, including my first EMG (electromyography), which tested for nerve and muscle disorders. Think cattle prod, because that's the best way to describe it. It was the first of many and actually the least painful.

The tests got more intense and unpleasant going forward. This first neurologist thought my body was trying to fight off a virus. I'll never forget sitting in his office, listening as he said, "I think a virus is attacking your body, and it could last anywhere from months to years for you to get better."

This vague diagnosis was literally mind-numbing to me. *Years? I'm thirty-one years old with two little kids and a full-time business. I don't have years to wait for this virus to pass, sir. Can't you do anything?*

Despite having no definitive answers, he was incredibly encouraging and willing to let me try antivirals for a little bit, which helped somewhat. Unfortunately, anything that gave me a bit of relief never lasted more than a month and then would gradually become ineffective. Whatever was attacking my body wasn't going to give up easily.

Five months into this strange illness, I felt like I was wandering around a deep forest where every possible path turned out to be a dead end.

{ *chapter four* }

DEEP BREATHS

"The peace I give is a gift the world cannot give.
So do not be troubled or afraid."

John 14:27b (NLT)

WHERE WE LIVE, SUMMER rolls in with waves
of heat and high humidity, along with a more relaxed schedule
because school's out. In the summer of 2012, I was still taking
on photoshoots, but I tried to keep a healthy balance of work
and play. Given my current situation, the idea of "play" was a
tough concept for me. I was graciously surrounded by some
amazing moms at school and church who loved me well,
especially during this time. They planned outings and playdates
and were sure to tell me where to meet them. All I had to do
was get the kids there. My friends would pack extra snacks for
my kids and make them lunches if I needed them to, which I
often did.

I was thankful for friends inviting me to the beach or the
park or wherever, really. Those ladies didn't know it then, but

those playdates kept me going. It would take everything in me to get to the playdate, so when I arrived, I usually just sat and talked about everything under the sun. Everything except my health. Because they knew. But they still loved me (and my big, bad pride) enough to avoid the topic.

I remember watching so much of life going by during these days. One particular day, as we sat on a picnic blanket in the park eating chicken salad sandwiches, I watched the kids run around, waving their arms effortlessly and skipping through the grass without a care in the world. I marveled at all that freedom and felt so thankful they had it. While I sat there, I noticed people's body language and animation when they talked. I would listen, but I would also wonder what it felt like to wave your arms in the air so freely or to make a casual gesture with your hand, without pain or even a thought.

Even in this strange fog, watching everything seem to float around me, I still had joy despite my circumstances. I took stock of the blessings in my life and, while I made a daily effort to push against how I felt physically, I wanted to actively acknowledge the truth of God's grace that my heart knew and believed. It's easy to get bogged down in how we feel physically and emotionally. How we feel on any given day can dictate everything, especially how we relate to other people. I clung to the fact that I serve a sovereign, all-knowing God and despite what I didn't know, He *did know*. He knows it all. I've always found comfort in how nothing surprises God. Trials and health crises and terrible events aren't problems for God to solve. Instead, the broken places are where His glory shines through. They're opportunities to draw near to Him and experience Him in ways we never have before.

At this point in my illness, I was aware of so many aspects

of God's character that I'd never experienced before. So in the middle of pain, nausea, confusion, and disillusionment was a deep sense of real peace. Even still, I spent a lot of time on my shower floor pleading with God. I asked for answers, because I thought that's what I needed. I begged God for something—anything—that could guide one of my doctors in a direction that would help me feel better. I was so confused that no one could figure out what was going on with me. It was in these moments that I realized I had to stop focusing on *what* and focus on *Who*.

Who could give me the strength to endure this confusion and extreme pain? *Who* could give me peace and joy? *Who* could comfort my family and friends?

God could. Not some diagnosis, but *God*.

One Sunday morning during that first year of being sick, we went around the room in our Sunday School class telling each other what we were thankful for. I was to Forbes's right, so my turn would come before his. My head swarmed. So many things to be thankful for. Where to start?

When it came around to me, I was speechless. Forbes just grabbed my hand and said, "We're thankful for this trial we're in because we have never felt closer to God." And there you have it. The hubs living and breathing one of my very favorite verses from one of my very favorite books in the Bible—James 1:2.

Consider it a sheer gift, friends, when tests and challenges come at you from all sides. You know that under pressure, your faith-life is forced into the open and shows its true colors. So don't try to get out of anything prematurely. Let it do its work so you become mature and well-developed, not deficient in any way. (MSG)

To be clear, we weren't some super righteous couple just smiling through our pain. We were two hurting people going through a really hard time. At the same time, we were fully believing that God was in it with us. The depth of God's presence and the spiritual growth we were experiencing in the midst of that valley was worth every moment of heartache and confusion.

It was a struggle to wake up each morning. Once I did, the weight I felt from what was going on with my body took full effect. I was several weeks into my newest symptom: shortness of breath. It felt like an elephant was sitting on my chest while I was trying to breathe through a clogged straw with weights attached.

I also started having these weird feelings in my chest, like a thud, as if my heart was dropping beats. Then it would suddenly slow down, which left me exhausted. My heart would drop beats and then beat at an abnormally low rate. And then, as fast as it had come on, it would simply go away. This symptom woke me up at night and took my breath during the day. Sometimes it would do this all day long, so that I felt like I was suffocating. Sometimes it would only happen at night. There was no rhyme or reason to it. The abnormal heartbeats came and went for a while and were so inconsistent that I decided to address my breathing issues first.

I met with a compassionate pulmonologist who was puzzled by my situation but willing to help. While examining me, she discovered a heart murmur. I'd never had a heart murmur before. I thought, with cautious hope, *Maybe this is it? Maybe this is the answer that we needed! Someone finally found something!* Now, don't think I'm crazy. I know it sounds odd for me to be excited about a heart murmur. But I was excited that one of my symptoms was going to be examined closer. While I was waiting in the exam room, I overheard the pulmonologist talking outside the door. "Something is going on," she said. "I'm sending her over for an echo today."

Soon as I heard the word *today*, I wanted to shout it out loud. TODAY! Who doesn't love immediate results? I wasted no time driving my sick self to the local hospital to get my first echocardiogram. It showed that a few things were off, which led me quickly to an appointment with a cardiologist.

When I say God is in every detail, He truly is. The pulmonologist sent me to a cardiologist, who just happened to have my mom and grandparents as patients. So he knew our family, which always helps. That said, I'm confident he would have had just as much compassion for me had he not known my family.

The cardiologist was intrigued by my symptoms. He was also helpful and genuinely encouraging, which I so desperately needed. Forbes and I were leaving for a friend's wedding the next day, so we asked about the risks of flying. The doctor looked at us and said, "Y'all need this trip. So here's what you'll need to do." He then recommended several things to help take care of my misbehaving heart for the flight. What a gift!

This doctor ended up being an advocate who refused to give up on me. When we got home from the wedding, he felt further examination was necessary and ordered a heart MRI. At that appointment, he encouraged me to go outside of my hometown to a bigger facility that could accommodate what had become my long list of symptoms. Actually, my neurologist and cardiologist agreed that being seen at a larger facility would be helpful.

So after my examination and the heart MRI, my inquisitive

and caring cardiologist paved the way for me to get an appointment at a much larger facility one state and several hours away.

Maybe My Heart Is the Problem

During the weeks between cardiology appointments and the MRI, I started wondering if all my issues were due to my heart. Not my physical heart. My spiritual one. I knew it was possible that psychological and emotional issues could manifest as physical issues. Besides, if we're honest, we all have problems with our spiritual heart. So I started to look inward.

I'd been through some difficult things as a child, and I knew God protected me through it all. I started asking Him if there were areas in my heart where I was harboring leftover baggage from those experiences. If we don't lose the junk in our hearts, we can't serve God wholeheartedly. After all, how can you serve God with your whole heart if half of it's holding onto things you won't surrender to Him?

I'm a very visual person. As such, I've always loved the image of laying my concern down at Jesus's feet. But here's the secret to doing that: I have to actually leave it there. If my thoughts continually go back to whatever "it" is, then I'm not really leaving "it" at His feet.

To learn more about what forces impact our hearts, I turned to Andy Stanley's book *Enemies of the Heart*.[3] What a great tool! In it, Stanley outlines the four forces that impact our hearts (jealousy, anger, greed, and guilt) and gives biblical truth to combat each one. What stood out to me was the importance of cleaning out my heart before going to bed. Stanley used this as an example with his own children.

At the end of the day, all those things I won't let go of or deal with get lugged around until I finally *do* deal with them. It could be something really small, seemingly insignificant. Think one tiny pebble in a rock wall. Every little piece, every moment of life, adds up. Before I know it, I'm middle-aged and confused about why I feel the way I do. Over the years, I've learned the hard way that neglecting to daily let go of those "little" things only means they become heavier and more difficult to toss out later. Seek the Lord, and I promise He'll show you what you need to let go of.

Stanley's book gave me the opportunity to take an honest look at my heart, and I was thankful for the time to do some real self-evaluation. I still use his book as a reference and a reminder when I'm feeling one of those forces he talks about. I never thought I struggled with anger, but I do get frustrated a lot, and—well, those emotions are definitely related. Anger doesn't always mean rage. Stanley points out, "Anger says, 'You owe me'." If I'm being honest, I felt like God owed me answers so I could get better. That sounds selfish as I write it, but it's true. Sure, I never felt full of rage, yelling at God while shaking my fists at the sky, but I did feel like I deserved answers. Then, I realized that I'm owed nothing. I'd already been given the greatest gift of all time: Jesus. He died for all my sins and gave me eternal life in Him.

In his study on Mark, Francis Chan puts it this way: "[Jesus] expects us to offer Him all of our lives; in return He offers us all of His."[4] Believing this gave me even more freedom to rest well where God had me and to surrender all of myself to Him. At the moment, I was in an uncomfortable wilderness with no relief in sight, but I had Jesus.

Bigger Places

In late July of that year, Forbes, my mom, and I headed to the Mayo Clinic, which had numerous specialists on staff. We spent a long and exhausting day seeing doctors, being examined, and answering questions. Some doctors were kind, others were not. Unfortunately, I ended up being seen by an insensitive neurologist. He told me he thought I had a central sensitization disorder, which is an umbrella term covering things like fibromyalgia and chronic fatigue syndrome. He agreed with me that neither of these very real syndromes truly applied to me but that I fit under the umbrella, mainly because my brain wasn't firing properly.

I was pretty dissatisfied with every word coming out of his mouth. I guess you could say I was, well, angry. The doctor suggested I start doing research and eating foods that helped my brain work at its highest capacity. Then as a bonus, he told me this wasn't an answer to everything. That more than one thing could be going on, so I shouldn't rule out other disorders in the future. I think he wanted me to understand that while he thought I had this particular disorder, it didn't mean something else hadn't also developed simultaneously.

I rode home in the backseat trying to figure out how I would explain to the people in my circle what the doctor said. At this point, all I knew was that I had a really vague diagnosis, which sort of explained things but also really didn't. I wanted to be careful how I said this, because even though the doctor confirmed something real was wrong with me, there were still many questions left unanswered.

I remember walking out of that medical center feeling a little less like the person who had walked in. Not long after, I plopped down on our couch and just stared at the carpet. I felt a pit in my stomach and acknowledged to myself that, even though that doctor's diagnosis might be right, I knew somehow that it wasn't really the answer to what was going on. Something specific had to be causing all the upheaval in my body. This sort of thing doesn't just happen out of nowhere. How can a perfectly healthy thirty-one-year-old runner suddenly develop issues with her brain firing unless something causes it? That's when I heard God's voice.

Okay, I know some of you are thinking, *What is this crazy lady talking about?* But I heard Him. I heard the Spirit whisper, "This is not a quick fix. You're going to get better, but you're going to have to hold on tight."

Obviously, I wasn't quite sure what that meant, but it gave me the peace I needed and the hope that I would get better in His time, not mine. Even though I felt some relief, it was still a tough pill to swallow. Let's be honest. God's timing is almost never ours. Do I hear an *amen?* And so I chose to focus on the *God-spoke-to-me!* part and press on.

I started doing extensive research on food that fueled and strengthened my brain. My local health food store became my favorite place. I began making all our food from scratch, determined to help this body I was stuck in, no matter what it took. It was around this time that someone suggested acupuncture. The concept was somewhat new to me, but I'd embraced enough of my circumstances to know that anything was worth a try. And with that, I entered a whole new world. Literally. Welcome to Chinese medicine, Sarah.

I'm kind of an all-or-nothing-type gal, so I jumped right in. By this point, most of my friends knew that I was struggling. Even if they thought I was totally off base, they just went with it. I tried to keep conversation about my expanding knowledge of how the body works to a minimum, because that can be annoying. But I was fascinated! I'd just finished the busy season with my business, so I had time to dive deep into the study of the body. I ended up going three times a week for acupuncture. It was no small expense, as far as time and money go. But I was totally in.

I was intrigued by this new (to me) way of healing the body and curious what else acupuncture could do. At one of my many appointments, as I waited in the small lobby, a young woman sat nearby with her baby, probably just a few months old at the time. I struck up a conversation. I was curious why she had her baby at an acupuncturist. The moment she opened her mouth, speaking with fervor and knowledge about the benefits of acupuncture, I was fascinated. She shared with me how her baby girl struggled with constant colic and that acupuncture seemed to help. Interesting! I told her how I wished I'd known about this when my son was a baby. I sure could have used some extra help with his cute, colicky self!

We chatted for a good ten minutes, mostly surface stuff. We introduced ourselves and she seemed to recognize my name, possibly because of my photography business. Her name was Kim, and she asked if I was there for a specific thing. I opened up to her about my mystery illness and even told her about a few of my symptoms, but I held a lot back. My pride wasn't going to fully divulge warts and all to this stranger I'd just met.

Pretty soon, my name was called. I stood up, said I hoped her baby got better and then commented, "It was super great to meet you, Kim." She said the same and wished me good luck with everything. And that was that. I went back into a little room where I laid on the exam table, feeling thankful for a conversation with a new acquaintance. Little did I know, this seemingly chance encounter was much more than it seemed at the time.

{ *chapter five* }

THE YEAR OF TRIALS

The deepest level of worship is
praising God in spite of pain,
thanking God during a trial,
trusting Him when tempted,
surrendering while suffering,
and loving him when he seems distant.[5]

Rick Warren

2013 WAS THE YEAR we referred to as the Year of Trials. And not just the specific trial we were going through with this health crisis, but also the year of trying new things.

With my newfound interest in nutrition and acupuncture, I decided to hire a nutritionist. Amy, a family friend, had just started her own nutrition business, so I was eager to get her involved in my health journey. Her involvement was exciting because it meant a new set of eyes to help navigate this mystery. What little I had gleaned from my own research, she quickly added to, or took away from, with real medical facts. Her knowledge was unreal. The first test she gave me was a food sensitivity test. I've always kind of looked at food as just a necessary means to an end. Fuel for the body. In the past year, however, eating had become something complicated. I had to be careful about what I ate because my stomach was so sensitive, and the consistency had to be just right or I would choke on it. No matter what I ate, I always felt terrible afterward. I attributed this to my body having to work so hard to function, which meant digesting food was just something else to wear it out. But what did I know?

I'll never forget sitting in the Target parking lot when Amy called with the results of my food sensitivity test .

"Sarah," she said, "holy cow, you are reacting to everything!"

Great, I thought. *What the heck does that mean?*

It meant the elimination diet was next on the agenda. Desperate to feel better, I jumped on to the next food-related bandwagon. Soon after, I hit a low point while sitting at a pizza restaurant having picked the kids up early from a half day of school. As the kids ate delicious, hot pizza, I ate a sad bowl of pinto beans and rice. Yes, you heard that right. Beans and rice were the two foods my body wasn't reacting to at the moment. And while beans and rice are just fine, when they're all you eat for weeks on end, it gets old. (Note: Pizza is my very, very favorite food. I mean, if you can't eat pizza, is life even worth living?) But I kept my chin up, ate my pinto beans, and determined to focus on the blessings all around me. Kids, without a care in the world, giggled over pizza with friends, thankfully unaware of how hard this all was for me. Despite everything, I was genuinely grateful in that moment to be present with my friends and our children.

I worked with Amy for many months after that. She was, in a word, amazing. She listened and researched, made phone calls on my behalf and answered every one of my questions with a prompt text. Not surprisingly, I had a lot of questions.

All the obvious things had been tested for so it was time to go rogue and try some out-of-the-box possibilities. Amy ordered blood tests and parasite tests, amongst others. She agreed with me that, ultimately, something specific had to be the cause of all the symptoms I was experiencing. Despite her efforts, after months of working with her, my gastrointestinal symptoms were back in full force. I did my best to adhere to a moderately strict diet, but the swallowing issues came back with a vengeance, and my diet became even more limited.

I decided to look for an internist again. My dearest college roommate Rachel, who is more like a sister to me, is married to Kevin, an internal medicine doctor outside of Atlanta. By this point, Kevin was fully informed about what I was dealing with and graciously offered medical counsel from afar. He looked over blood work and handled several emotional calls and texts from me. He suggested I make an appointment with a doctor he worked with previously.

That day, I got home and told Forbes that I was really excited about my next doctor's visit. I explained that Kevin had given me the name of a new internist and I had an appointment with him in two weeks. Forbes said that was great and then asked what his name was. When I told him it was Dr. B, he spun around.

"That's my doctor!" Forbes said as he laughed.

My response? "Well, thanks for nothing. Kevin gets the credit on this!"

Dr. B was a godsend. To this day, he still manages all my health shenanigans. Initially, Forbes and I went to him to discuss my mystery illness, but also for advice on my digestive issues. Not long before, I called Forbes at work one evening. I asked him to come home early, because I was on the floor with stomach pain so intense I could barely see or form words. That was the night Forbes said enough is enough.

We talked with Dr. B and he ordered blood work as every other doctor had, but he offered something else: compassion and hope. I couldn't help but think, *Third time's the charm! Little does he know, he's stuck with me now!* After several meetings and a referral to a gastroenterologist, Dr. B talked with us about what happens to the body and brain after months of pain and sleeplessness. He kindly persuaded me to try some antidepressant meds.

"I don't think this is an issue for you," he said, "but this is a hard thing to go through, and medication may help."

So, with my tail between my legs, I took the meds. Five weeks later, my swallowing was worse than ever.

I waited desperately for the appointment with the gastroenterologist Dr. B referred me to. Unfortunately, it ended up being less than ideal. The doctor looked at me skeptically as I explained my symptoms, and I could tell he wasn't really listening. It was almost as if he was looking straight through me as I talked. While there, he performed an EGD, a quick procedure that looks down the esophagus to the stomach to see what's going on. Biopsies were taken, but nothing looked abnormal. All the biopsies came back—you guessed it—normal. I'm pretty surprised rage didn't take over at this point. The stomach aches I experienced at times were totally debilitating, so it was discouraging, to say the least, to not get any answers.

I think my determination to keep going came out of pure desperation. With no real solutions on the horizon, Forbes and I decided to see a new neurologist. We were blessed yet again to have a doctor friend of ours get us in for an appointment relatively quickly. We had no problem with my other neurologist, but it felt like a new set of eyes was needed. My first encounter with this new doctor was like most. He had the same curiosity and desire to dig deeper into my illness. It was oddly interesting to watch and I almost felt a bit of pride that my mystery health issue genuinely challenged each doctor's knowledge base. I must say, however, that this doctor gave it a real go.

In a six-week time period, I had a spinal tap, another brain MRI, a spine MRI, as well as tests for lead and mold. You name it, he ran the test on me. Everything was normal except for my brain MRI, which showed white spots on my brain, something they told me was indicative of migraines.

Hmmm, that's strange, I thought.

I could only remember having three migraines in my life. This conclusion didn't settle with me, so I just tucked it into my back pocket, hoping it would be useful at a later time. Even so, the day the nurse called to tell me my results, I was pretty adamant that I didn't have migraines. She was equally adamant that I was wrong. I got that a lot, so I just went with it.

August arrived and almost every symptom that had waxed and waned over the last eighteen months converged on me with intensity. My nausea and stomach pain were nearly unbearable. My hands folded in like claws. It took unbelievable effort to take photos. I had to concentrate hard to make my hands work properly, all while trying to get toddlers and babies to smile at me.

My swallowing was so impaired that by the time summer ended, I was on a completely liquid diet, which meant I just pureed everything. All I'd learned in the past about nutrition became extremely helpful at this point. I ate healthy soups and added cooked kale to almost everything I blended to get the nutrients I needed. But the key was consistency. If it was too thick, it would get stuck. Too thin, and I would choke on it. I would even choke on water. I had to hold my head a certain way and concentrate when I drank to avoid choking. I drank thickened broth and ate more Luigi ice cups than I care to share just to soothe the painful soreness in my throat muscles.

Since I'm already divulging too much, I'll admit that if I leaned over after drinking water, it would come out of my nose. Envision that while taking baby photos on all fours during a photo shoot. Yeah, not great. AT ALL!

I remember one particular weekend when my issues with swallowing became glaringly obtrusive in my social life. Once a year, Forbes, myself, Elizabeth and her husband, Chris, enjoy a fun-filled weekend at our alma mater, the University of Georgia. We head to Athens, Georgia, one of our favorite cities, to shop, eat, and cheer on our beloved Bulldogs. That particular year, we discussed canceling, but I insisted we go. I knew getting away would be good for all of us. However, I have a bad habit of ignoring the obvious. I don't do it all the time, but it happened a lot while I was sick.

I'd been on liquids for a while at this point, but being the non-foodie that I am, I didn't think it would hinder our trip. Turns out, when you're surrounded by foodies, it matters. One evening, we searched up and down our favorite streets for a restaurant that served soup. I was exhausted from the walking. I wanted to give up, but they wouldn't.

We finally found a restaurant with a minimal wait that served soup. The waitstaff let me sit in the only chair available as we waited. As we sat down to order, I requested the only soup they had on the menu.

The server quickly replied, "I'm so sorry, but we are out of soup tonight." I thought Forbes, Elizabeth, and Chris were all going to cry.

"No problem!" I said.

Looking down at the menu, I saw they had cheese-covered fries. Desperate to keep things cool and not ruin our night, I ordered them. I hated the attention being on me. I secretly cringed at my unhealthy choice and hoped I could mash them up enough to get them down with a swig of hot tea. I felt like a ninety-year-old stuck in a thirty-two-year-old's body. I would have been fine sitting there just drinking water, but it mattered to them, which made it matter to me.

When the swallowing issue got so bad I couldn't swallow pills anymore, Dr. B helped me wean off the antidepressant medication. The pills weren't really doing anything anyway, so I needed to stop taking them since they were getting stuck, too. He asked the gastro doctor to get involved again, and this time the gastro ordered what today is still the worst test I have ever had: the esophageal manometry test.

By the grace of God, Forbes got called to a meeting he couldn't miss, so my mom escorted me to this appointment. Forbes and my mom had both been present at almost every one of my appointments, and I cannot imagine how exhausted they must have been by now. Neither of them ever said a word or complained. But it was divine intervention that Forbes was able to sit this one out.

For those who are unfamiliar with the esophageal manometry test, it works like this: a weighted tube is shoved up your nose and down your throat. Then you swallow so it can measure the function of the throat muscles. Prior to this test, I'd been poked and prodded a lot, but this was next level stuff.

It was also one of the most humbling experiences of my life. Bless that sweet lady who performed the test.

During the test, I threw up all over myself six times. There was nothing I could do to keep it from happening. On top of the vomit, the pain was unreal. It felt like she was cutting my neck open with a knife and then asking me to swallow. WOWZERS!

The memory of that day still gets to me. Even though my husband had witnessed a lot up to that point, no man needs to see his wife vomiting uncontrollably all over herself. My mom, as usual, was a rock star. She kept as quiet as she could while holding the vomit tub that I skillfully missed every time. She knew nothing she could say could make the situation any better, and I know her mama heart hurt for me.

Despite the awfulness of that whole experience, it was helpful. This horrific test did more than hurt and humble me. It revealed that I did, in fact, have a real issue. This insight gave us some hope as it offered more information for the doctors to work with.

More tests were run—a gastric-emptying test, abdominal scans, and another swallow study. In the second swallow study, I met with a speech/swallow specialist who was incredibly compassionate. She taught me some tricks to use and provided more education on liquid nutrition. I'd hope that every step we took and every person we met along the way brought us another step closer to some kind of resolution.

At my second swallow test, the possibility of a feeding tube was brought up. Throughout the seven months of having serious swallowing issues and only consuming liquids, it had been suggested several times. But I firmly refused. I wouldn't get a feeding tube without knowing what was wrong with me. If I had to endure a feeding tube, I wanted a reason for it.

Soon after, I experienced a sudden, noticeable decline. I was blacking out—a lot. So my cardiologist jumped back into the picture. He was very kind, teaching me what to do when I started to black out so that I wouldn't injure myself. During this time, muscular sclerosis (MS) and similar illnesses were mentioned, but nothing that could be definitively diagnosed was showing up. ALS and cancer were also popping up in conversations with my doctors, but only as vague possibilities.

We were fortunate to get yet another doctor involved who knew our family and had heard about my health crisis. (It was pretty safe to say it was a crisis at this point.) He and his amazing nurse were encouraging. After his examination, he concluded that the vague diagnoses being considered might not be totally off base. It definitely appeared to either be a hard-to-diagnose MS case, ALS, or a hidden cancer causing a neoplastic syndrome, which just meant the cancer could be causing all the issues I was experiencing.

I'd had most of my organs scanned by this point, so cancer was a less likely diagnosis than the other two possibilities. This doctor got me an appointment with an ALS specialist a few weeks later at Emory Hospital's neurology department. I left that appointment feeling heavy. In one visit, the doctor validated what other doctors suspected. The thought of those awful diagnoses in my overly optimistic mind was difficult to process. I was in a complete funk the rest of the day as those previously ruled-out diagnoses were now very valid possibilities.

The September appointment at Emory felt like our last hope. We believed we had exhausted all our other options. Forbes, my mom and dad, and I traveled the four hours to Emory and then sat patiently in the waiting room. I couldn't help but feel like my second home was a waiting room.

Initially, I was seen by a young resident who was the assistant, or in actuality, the gatekeeper to this great doctor we thought we had come to see. After the assistant's examination, she said I definitely did not have ALS. But she wasn't sure what was going on with me. She was less than compassionate, which made me want to cry as I listened to her. It was like watching my balloon of hope slowly deflate before my eyes. I wanted to melt into the table, a puddle of disappointment.

Don't get me wrong, we were *elated* with the non-ALS confirmation, but we also had pits in our stomachs. The assistant ordered another test for the following morning to make sure I wasn't having seizures while I was sleeping. What we thought was a pivotal appointment was over in a blink.

The next morning, they performed an EEG, which required them to hook wires to my head so they could see my brain activity. Forbes was allowed in the room for this one. I looked ridiculous with the wires everywhere, so despite the heaviness of the situation, we took the opportunity to laugh. We even sent a few silly photos to my sister and friends. This test felt like our last available option. Afterward, we drove back home and waited for the results.

There were a number of songs throughout the previous eighteen months that I had claimed as being "for me." As a matter of fact, a year prior, when we embarked on our first out-of-state medical trip, Elizabeth made me a playlist with various worship songs. Worship was my jam. It was a way to keep my thoughts off myself and on the One who made me.

Like Psalm 91:2 says, "The Lord is my refuge and my fortress and I will trust in Him." The lyrics of John Waller's song "While I'm Waiting" became ingrained in my thoughts:

While I'm waiting
I will serve You
While I'm waiting
I will worship
While I'm waiting
I will not faint
I'll be running the race
Even while I wait[6]

I also found an excerpt from a blog post by a well-known Bible teacher that gave me much hope about the waiting period I was in. Read her words carefully:

Before God moves suddenly, we will wait. Waiting for answers is a fact of life—nobody gets out of it. So the question is not if we'll wait, but rather how we'll wait. We know the word "wait" means "to expect" or "to look for." But remember, it also means "to serve"—just like a waiter waits on your table at a restaurant. Our act of waiting isn't supposed to be spent sitting around passively hoping that something will happen sometime soon. Once we've asked God to answer a question or solve a problem, we need to be eagerly awaiting His answer. We need to be serving actively, aggressively and expectantly. . . . In many cases this waiting period actually serves as a time of preparation for the answer. If God answered right away, many of us would be ill-prepared to handle His solution.[7]

Waiting is just part of life. What we do *while* we're waiting prepares us for where GOD takes us next. Basically, how we wait matters, and I knew in this moment that I wanted to wait well.

When Two or More Gather

As you are well aware of by now, God kept showing me I had to deal with my pride. In the early stages of my illness, when it became obvious that something major was going on but we didn't know what, I shut a lot of people out. I couldn't put into words what was happening, so I thought if I just didn't talk about it, I could pretend it wasn't happening. However, there were six friends at our church who loved me enough to take matters into their own hands. After convincing me to meet with them on Wednesday nights for prayer, they offered me space to vent and to be honest with my feelings, my frustrations, and the guilt that I couldn't be the mom I wanted to be.

During these gatherings, my sweet friend Brooke spoke truth to that crippling guilt I felt and boldly reminded me that conviction comes from the Lord, but guilt comes from Satan. That was her subtle but loving way of firmly saying *no* to the lies I was allowing Satan to tell me and her exhortation to embrace the truths of God's Word. She reminded me that God was daily giving me all the strength I needed to operate in the capacity I needed to operate. That's when I realized I had to lower my expectations of myself. I'm not sure why it took me crying and being real with that small group of friends to finally realize that, but it did.

In Jennie Lusko's book *Fight to Flourish*, she puts into words why those prayer meetings were so significant.

When we bring others into our pain, we position ourselves to receive the wisdom, insight, and a different perspective than we would have gained otherwise.[8]

That raw time of sitting on the floor as friends laid hands

on me and prayed over me with not a dry eye in the room was telling. It told of Christ's love for me. Of my friends' love for me. What I was going through was hard to watch for those who loved me, but we knew there was purpose in it, even if we couldn't understand it. Jesus understood it and He wasn't going to let any of it go to waste.

Sadly, it was a year into my illness before I was okay with my name being added to prayer lists at our church and other local churches. It's no coincidence that when the fervent prayers started, answers followed! I had people praying for me in New York, Georgia, South Carolina, Colorado, Florida, and beyond. Some people were fasting and others were waking up at 3 a.m. to pray. Friends were a constant encouragement, consistently emailing and texting to say they were praying. It was all incredibly humbling.

Psalm 73:26 says, "My flesh and my heart may fail, but God is the strength of my heart and my portion forever." I've read this verse many times throughout my life, but I now know what it truly means. *The Lord is my portion.* He gives me exactly what I need to get through every moment of every single day. So often, I get ahead of myself, focusing on what I want, and forget that simple truth.

He is always enough.

{ chapter six }

THE WORST THREE MONTHS

For now we see in a mirror dimly,
but then face to face.
Now I know in part; then I shall know fully,
even as I have been fully known.

I Corinthians 13:12

BY OCTOBER OF 2013, I finally relinquished a little of my prideful self-sufficiency and consented to an email list being put together for friends and family who wanted to know what was going on and how they could pray more specifically for me. I still hadn't received a diagnosis or gotten any better. In fact, many of my symptoms had gotten worse. Even so, I was overwhelmingly aware of God's nearness and His powerful work in me.

There was a constant stream of encouraging phone calls, texts and prayers from so many, which was truly amazing. We had friends call friends who called in favors to help us connect with specific doctors, which was the most humbling experience.

With each of those phone calls, of course, came more waiting, which by now you would think I'd be used to, but I wasn't.

After numerous emails, a few long phone calls and loads of records passed back and forth, I had appointments scheduled with three neurologists, all specialists in different aspects of their field. Two were located in Atlanta and one in Charleston, South Carolina, and the appointments were spread over a three-day period that October. We could make a movie about how those appointments came about, which involved God mobilizing an army of people to help us. It was astonishing to be in the midst of it all, watching the pieces fall into place over and over.

While I was grateful for all the effort it took our precious friends to make these appointments happen for me, I began to worry about the repercussions of receiving three different doctors' perspectives almost simultaneously. What would it look like to follow the advice of multiple doctors at the same time, all of whom were located miles away from us?

I prayed constantly about this. After a conversation with my dad about prayer, I wondered if I knew how to pray at all. It wasn't that I didn't think God was hearing my prayers. I just didn't seem to be getting any answers. Was I even doing it right?

Around the same time I was agonizing over my multiple appointment situation, my grandmother was attending a dinner for cancer survivors in her hometown. Every year, a portion of the funds raised at this event for cancer research are donated to Emory in Atlanta, and an Emory doctors comes to receive the donation on behalf of the center.

After the dinner that evening, my grandmother had a feeling (hello, Holy Spirit) that she was supposed to talk to the doctor who received the donation. Tears in her eyes, she boldly walked up to him.

"My granddaughter is very sick and we're running out of options," she said. "Could you help us?"

She then described my symptoms, and he gave her his email address in response. He said he wasn't sure if he could help, but he would love to try.

This doctor and I emailed back and forth multiple times. Each time, he would ask a few more questions in an attempt to determine how he could help. I was encouraged by his quick replies to my emails and his offer to connect me with whichever doctor I wanted. I was pretty determined to see the well-renowned neurologist at Emory who specializes in ALS. For some reason, I believed ALS couldn't be completely ruled out unless this doctor physically saw me. However, the doctor I'd been emailing with had a better plan. His solution was even better than I could have hoped.

One Thursday morning, feeling desperate, I decided to be quiet during my prayer time. Instead of my usual non-stop talking and pleading, I focused intently on Psalm 46:10: "Be still, and know that I am God."

As I sat down with the sincere goal of being completely still and quiet, something told me to reach for my phone, which was the total opposite of what I had just resolved to do. I couldn't help but laugh at myself. *I'm trying so hard to be still with the Lord and yet here I am, reaching for my phone, the source of every possible distraction.*

A moment later, the phone rang. On the other end of the line was the most cheerful, calming voice I'd ever heard.

"Is this Sarah?"

I knew immediately this was an important conversation. I was speaking to the head administrator of the diagnostic center at Emory Hospital in Atlanta, which I didn't know existed.

After an encouraging forty-minute conversation, she said she would help me! The center she worked with employed a team of doctors from all specializations who consulted on hard-to-diagnose cases. Basically, instead of going to a dozen different specialists in a dozen different locations, they were all grouped together on the same property, allowing them to discuss ideas with their team after meeting with a patient.

It was a dream situation for someone like me, who had multi-systemic issues. Tears stung my eyes when she said they could see me on the exact day I already had a neurologist appointments scheduled. It felt like a direct answer to my prayer, another reminder that God is in *every* detail.

The "appointment" at Emory's diagnostic center was actually a week-long appointment, which meant I saw multiple specialists instead of just one. After that phone call, I canceled my other three neurologist appointments. The angst I'd been feeling over those melted away.

I thought back over the past few days and weeks—the conversations I'd had with Forbes, my friends, and my parents about which appointment to keep. Now I had an answer: none of them. I had another appointment instead.

Why was it always so hard for me to trust that God was taking care of things? It reminded me of a blog post my sweet friend emailed to me not long before this about our expectations of life and how, like impatient children, we're always asking questions, wanting to know what's next. And God, our patient Father, simply reminds us, *"YOU'LL SEE!"*

The post read:

. . . [S]o often, I ply my Heavenly Father with anxious questions . . .

What are you doing next, Lord?
Where are you taking me?
When will this be over?

I don't just ask these questions once. I ask them over and over. And more often than not, God replies with the same answer I give [my son], *"You'll see."*

To be honest, I don't like that answer any more than [my son] does. And yet when I grumble about God's response, I fail to see the massive mercy behind it. *"You'll see"* is a promise. A glorious promise, secured for me at the cross! I will see! Because I have been adopted into God's family through the atoning death of Jesus Christ on my behalf, I will one day see God.

See what kind of love the Father has given to us, that we should be called children of God; and so we are. The reason why the world does not know us is that it did not know Him. Beloved, we are God's children now, and what we will be has not yet appeared; but we know that when He appears, we shall be like Him, because we shall see Him as He is (John 3:1-2 ESV).[9]

Friend, you *will* see. But, it means being patient in the waiting. And as we all know, waiting is always the hardest part of anything. It's in that place where we have to cling tight to Isaiah 55:8: "'For My thoughts are not your thoughts, neither are your ways My ways,' declares the Lord." As my dad loves to remind me, God's ways are *way better* than ours!

I can't help but marvel at how over a four-week period, three significant appointments were made and canceled, my grandmother attended that timely dinner, and now I had this incredible opportunity to be seen at Emory's diagnostic center, which was a direct result of my grandmother's obedience to God's Spirit.

It's important to know that regardless of the hard place you're stuck in or the trial you're slogging through, none of it is wasted. God redeems and gives value to even the worst of circumstances for His glory and our good. But we need to be ready and available for that moment when God chooses to move.

My grandmother survived breast cancer thirty years before this particular dinner for cancer survivors. Thirty years is a long time to wait for redemption, but God graciously allowed her to see a difficult chapter in her story be redeemed in my story. She wouldn't have been at that dinner had she not been diagnosed with cancer all those years before. And I wouldn't have benefited from that redemption if she hadn't been ready and available to hear from God's Spirit.

Think about the hard thing you're walking through right now. Consider with hope that it has purpose in God's sovereignty. He will use it for good.

Even Bigger Place, Even More Tests

Finally, the day we'd been holding our breaths for arrived. When we arrived at the center, we were a little stunned at how impressive it all was. Forbes, my parents, and I walked in, each of us in awe that we were here.

To begin, we were interviewed together as a family and then separately. I knew there was some real concern for my psychological well-being at this point, so, in order to be thorough, they dug in deep with my family. Questions like, *Is it possible that someone could actually be poisoning Sarah?* and *Does Sarah like getting attention from others?* were asked. Thankfully, I wasn't present for those conversations, which was probably to prevent me and my opinions from getting in the way of honest answers.

Before we left for this trip, many people were fasting and praying for us. Everyone knew that a lot weighed on this opportunity and that it would include long, exhausting hours with lots of questions and lots of tests. Elizabeth sent me a list of Bible verses that focused on hope and the promises of God. I printed the list out, folding it in half and then in half again the other way. Every time I sat alone in a room waiting for a doctor or a test to be performed, I pulled out that little folded-up paper and prayed those verses over and over. I read and reread those verses as I sat on the bench outside the center, waiting to be picked up for my next appointment. They helped alleviate the fears that would creep in the second I let my guard down. They even helped the feelings of hopelessness I had, wondering if this would ever end.

I spent the first week at the center going to all sorts of tests and meetings with a variety of specialists. My condition piqued many of their interests. After that initial week, we headed home, only to make the four-hour drive again when another doctor at the diagnostic center had an idea and wanted to test something.

One of the greatest gifts of those trips was that my dear friend, Rachel, lived nearby and would come to see me, eating a meal with us when she could. Well, she would eat with Forbes or my mom, while I sipped on my chicken broth. It was so fun to have her visit, because she always had great stories about her kids or life. In that time between doctor appointments, she helped me feel like a normal person. Looking back now, those lunch dates got me through some really long days. Sometimes I was too sick to even think about my schedule or tell Rachel the right time to meet us, so she would communicate with Forbes or my mom instead. If it had been left to me, I would have just said I didn't know when to meet. Keeping all the dates, times, and locations in mind took too much brain power. I so appreciated her persistence in our friendship.

The biggest hurdle I had to overcome was that every doctor I saw was adamant that once I hit a certain point, in order to move forward with treatment and more testing, I needed to meet with a psychologist. To say I was furious would be an understatement. However, the fight in me was dwindling, and I knew agreeing to this was a means to an end. I also knew that I was not insane, so what did I have to lose?

I remember the tightness in my chest and butterflies in my stomach on the drive to my psychologist appointment. I purposefully left this appointment off the email updates I'd been sending. I wanted this one to slip through the cracks, to go unnoticed. As a result, I only confessed to a few people what "test" I was having on this trip.

The psychologist who saw me was a compassionate and intriguing man. At this point, my faith and my relationship with Christ had exploded with growth, so how could I not talk about it? I told myself—and asked God for help—to not shed *one* tear in this meeting. There was still some pride borrowing inside me, and I didn't want to appear weak. Even worse, insane! I was there to prove I was mentally stable. But as I shared with the psychologist all I'd learned through my journey and how, even though this was the hardest thing I had ever gone through, I'd never felt closer to God, the tears started rolling.

He asked a few questions, including, "Why are you crying right now?"

There was my opportunity to share my faith. And crazy as

it sounds, I shared the gospel with that psychologist right then and there, during my psych evaluation.

I remember Forbes's facial expression when the door opened, revealing his extreme relief that it was over. An hour into our drive, we got a call confirming that I was, in fact, completely sane. The director related the gist of what the psychologist's had to say, which was that "She's a very strong, well-grounded young lady of faith, and I hope that you all can get to the bottom of her illness soon."

Boom!

The relief I felt after that was unreal. Forbes turned to me. "What did you think they would say?" he asked.

I told him at this point, I didn't know what to think. I only knew God was sovereign, which was what I told the psychologist.

The one symptom that showed up the most out of all the tests they ran was the swallowing issue. Every test confirmed that there was definitely a problem.

To try to find an answer, I was sent to one of the top gastroenterologists in Atlanta, who also specializes in movement disorders. After my second EGD in five months, the gastroenterologist confirmed that there was significant damage to my esophagus that hadn't been there five months before. Most importantly, he stretched my narrowing esophagus all the way down. In a matter of weeks, I could eat solid food again!

The doctor met with us after the procedure to explain what he'd done. I was still pretty drugged, so Forbes did all the note taking and question asking. He told us that he had no idea what was causing the swallowing issue or how long the stretching would last. It could be a week or a year. Only time would tell.

About a week later, the diagnostic center called and said that although my symptoms were real, they could find no explanation for them, and they would see me again in six months.

There was no hole deep enough for me to climb into. My heart throbbed in my ears, and I felt the darkness of despair like I had not experienced before. I distinctly remember that I was working at my desk when I got the call and how, without warning, intense desperation and grief swept over me like a wave. *What? There's no way!* I was unwilling to accept that I had to wait six more months to see if my condition would get worse.

At this point, Audrey and Warren were six and three years old, and they really needed their mom to get better. In this dark moment was frustration, anger, and what felt like deep embarrassment. I'm not sure why, other than that I felt like I'd dragged my family, friends, and church through this long ordeal with me. And all for nothing, it seemed. All the traveling, all the babysitters, all the friends bringing meals and helping shuffle kids around. I felt that so many had been on this journey with me, and I'd let them down. It wasn't until much later that I understood the intense emotion I felt wasn't embarrassment. It was shame.

I called my mom to tell her the news, and she thought I was kidding. She asked how it was even possible. I said, "I don't know, but I don't want to talk about it. I just wanted you to know."

I wanted to shut everyone out BIG time at that point. I was done with it all. If I could have, I would have locked myself away and tossed the key.

I know now every single doctor I saw and every single test I went through was necessary to get me to where I am today. I'm thankful for all the doctors, who even though they were puzzled and unable to offer an actionable solution, eliminated some frightening diagnoses like cancer, MS, and ALS. I still sincerely appreciate their tenacity and determination to help me find answers.

But without a diagnosis, the journey continued. And while I didn't have much fight left in me at that moment, I knew God was still in it with me. In fact, He was becoming more real to me with each day that passed.

{ *chapter seven* }

CLOSED DOORS & OPEN DOORS

Rest in the Lord, and wait patiently.
The Lord knows the days of the upright.

Psalm 37:7, 18 (KJV)

WITH SO MANY THINGS happening in our lives, it took a while to realize it was time to deal with the elephant in the room. No, not my illness. One of the sources of my greatest pride and joy: my business. This hard realization slowly began to dawn on me during the weeks leading up to the diagnostic center appointments, and I knew that something had to change.

I fretted constantly about what I was going to do about my beloved photography business. The strategy and brain power required to maneuver my camera at photoshoots was diminishing by the day. More significantly, the pain that holding my camera caused was becoming unbearable, and my ability to carry my camera bag was long gone. October was peak shoot season, the time when everyone wants family photos for Christmas cards and gifts, and I had a full calendar lined up. I took my job very seriously and was honored that each client continued to let me capture their growing families. I felt like part of so many of those families, so not only could I not let them down, I genuinely didn't want to. I wanted to see all my favorite people and their sweet babies again.

Forbes and I talked about how many sessions I would need to take care of everyone before I could finally stop working. *Ugh.* I shuddered at the thought of stopping. I pored over the calendar, made numerous phone calls, and talked with clients about moving their sessions so I could do back-to-back shoots, which would help me to finish sooner. Once I made the mid-October appointment at the diagnostic center, my goal became finishing my photoshoots before then. That would allow me six weeks to turn around the edited photos and get them back to my clients—not my normal process. Typically during busy season, I would do a shoot and then have the edited photos back to my client within a week. Since everything else in life had been forced to change, so did the way I ran my business.

All my clients, recognizing I was in a pretty fragile state, were *so* understanding and compassionate toward me. And I needed every bit of it. I diligently took my pureed kale smoothies and chicken broth with me to every shoot to ensure I had the energy to take the best photos I could. It was grueling, but I was determined to finish every last one.

This was about the time that I realized nothing nutritionally was really helping or hurting me, so why not bring back my beloved coffee? I did, and my old friend caffeine helped get me through all those shoots.

The decision to close my business was one of the hardest I'd had to make so far. At some point, I fervently declared to Forbes that there was no way I would lose my business and everything I worked so hard to accomplish to a disease that didn't even have a name yet! But it was inevitable.

As hard as it was, the fact that I physically couldn't do it anymore oddly softened the blow . . . a little bit. I really struggled with the aftermath of this decision, though. For so long, I'd been the trusted, go-to family photographer with boundless energy and zest for life and now, what was I? Some sick person with no answers who was losing her business. This moment was when I really started to struggle with my identity. Not only did I not recognize the washed-out, gaunt face in the mirror, but who was I if I couldn't take photos anymore?

I also realized it was time to confess to Forbes that my memory was failing so badly that I couldn't remember driving places. We decided the safest thing was for me to stop driving, especially with the kids. That was just one more mom duty I grieved losing. One afternoon, after I wasn't driving anymore, Elizabeth drove me to Lifeway. There, I picked up a Mark Driscoll book called *Who Do You Think You Are?* I'd read about this book online and thought it could be helpful for what I was going through. It turned out that it was a great resource, providing biblical truths to help explain the biblical concept of identity in Christ. It forced me to do a lot of soul searching and deep diving to work through this idea.

In his book, Driscoll highlights the book of Ephesians, specifically chapters 1 and 2, which describe so eloquently what it means to be a child of God. What resonated most with me in this study was the identity we have as God's children. Because we belong to the Father, we are saints (1:1), blessed (1:3), chosen (1:4), adopted (1:5), redeemed (1:7), forgiven (1:7), sealed (1:13), loved (2:4) and saved (2:5).[10]

If you struggle to wrap your head around who you are

down deep, take comfort in these verses in Ephesians. Maybe something you felt was an important part of your identity has been taken from you and you don't know how to move on. Maybe it's a relationship, a spouse, a job, or even a physical part of your body that's been lost. No matter what *it* is, it can be difficult when those things can't define you anymore. It's easy to let something consume us so quickly we don't realize we've made it a part of our identity until it's removed. But everything we need to tell us who we are, God has already revealed to us in His Word. If you struggle with your identity, dive into Ephesians. Let God tell you about your true identity in Him.

Despite how I felt, clients still needed their cards and photos in time for Christmas. So I stayed at my desk, listening to music and cranking out edited photos like a robot.

I've been pretty honest here about how I felt physically and emotionally, but you may be wondering what I looked like on the outside. I looked pretty rough. I was frail and underweight, and I kept hearing that the usual twinkle in my eye was gone. Jesus, coffee, and make-up go a long way, but those who know me could see right through the caffeine and lipstick. I desperately wanted our life to look as normal as possible, especially for our kids. But there was nothing normal about our lives. Every meal, every outing, every ponytail that needed tying, every glass of milk that needed pouring felt impossible, and the weight of the unknown Forbes and I carried was overwhelming. Still, Forbes and I did our best to do life in a way that felt like us. Keeping things going felt important and somehow life-giving to our weary souls.

It was almost Thanksgiving. Every other year, our families take turns hosting everyone for the holiday. My in-laws live four hours away, and Forbes's sister's family lives in Colorado. This particular year, it was my in-laws' turn to host, so we planned to visit Colorado. There was a lot of excitement for the upcoming trip, but also a lot of stress. I was frantically wrapping up most of my photography work before we left, but when the call from the diagnostic center came, everything came to a screeching halt. When I heard they couldn't make a diagnosis, it was like a speeding car slammed into a glass wall, throwing shattered glass everywhere. Trying to work while also picking up the shards of my hope created so many emotions going into this trip.

Will it all just make me feel worse?

The thought crossed our minds by now that this might be our last opportunity to do something like this as a family. We had no idea what the future held in light of my health. Then in the midst of working, packing, and managing a roller coaster of emotions, I noticed a new Facebook message.

At the time, I was using Facebook more than at any point in my entire life because of my business. However, I still wasn't all that familiar with receiving messages there. Assuming it was someone reaching out to book a session, I clicked on the message, already forming my response: *I'm so sorry, but at this time I have no more open spots for 2013.* Before I could finish that response in my head, I started reading the message.

It wasn't someone asking about a session. It was Kim. My acupuncturist waiting-room friend I'd met almost a year prior.

Her message read something like this,

Hey, Sarah, this is Kim. I'm not sure where you are in your health journey, but I noticed when you walked away from me that day that your leg was dragging. I've recently been on my own health journey and watched this documentary on Lyme disease and it made me think of you.

Okay now, wait a minute! What? I met this girl *one* time. In a waiting room. She had NO idea where I was on my health journey. For all she knew, I was doing great and skydiving in my free time. She warned me that the documentary[11] was intense, so I may not want to watch it all at once. (Note: I would never actually skydive because I don't do heights!)

Intrigued, I carried my laptop upstairs and started watching the video while I stuffed sweaters into my bag for the trip. Forbes had the kids somewhere so it was just me, myself, and this laptop.

Kim wasn't joking. The documentary was intense. I watched it in three pieces, but mostly because of my mom duties and the fact that we were getting ready to leave town. Once I was halfway through the movie, I knew this was it. Lyme disease was the mystery illness I'd been dealing with for nearly two years. But my next thought was, *How in the world am I going to get someone to diagnose this?*

I'd already been tested for it several times with negative results. But the documentary explained that the CDC test for it was not strong enough to detect Lyme, especially if someone has had it for a long time. I found this so hard to wrap my brain around. We live in such a technologically advanced world. How could we not have a test to detect such an awful disease?

Questions swarmed like flies at a picnic. I prayed, "God, I know this is what I have, please give us wisdom if this is something you want us to pursue." Soon after, I exchanged numbers with Kim and she became part of my health journey. Honestly, her reaching out that day changed the course of my journey in *so* many ways.

To give you a little background on Kim, she battled random, debilitating symptoms on and off for ten years before discovering Lyme disease was the culprit. After the birth of her second child, the culmination of her symptoms came to a head. Interestingly, her daughters' pediatrician suggested she get tested for Lyme disease.

Kim compares our experiences with the disease as her going down a spiral staircase of symptoms, while I abruptly fell through a hole in the floor. Despite being relative strangers to one another, Kim unselfishly shared her wealth of holistic health knowledge with me and over time became a beloved friend.

After watching the documentary she shared, I allowed myself to feel a tiny sliver of hope in this possible answer. But all the while I knew my ultimate hope was in Jesus and if this was something to pursue, He would guide us.

A New Symptom Appears

We traveled to Colorado a few days after I watched the video. We love any opportunity to spend time with family, so we purposely focused on what was in front of us and tried not to talk about this new possibility we were about to pursue. Forbes was intrigued, but still a bit skeptical, so we continued to pray.

Seeing our family and the beauty of Colorado was exactly what we needed! Our family lives right outside of Denver, but we rented a house in Breckenridge for part of our visit. It would be a fun week for cousins to giggle, play in the snow, sled, and eat lots of good food. I was starting to introduce more and more solid food into my diet each day, but still had to be careful. Certain foods still caused severe stomach aches.

Despite the pain and feeling terrible, I managed to have some fun. It was such a relief to be away and have a distraction from all the hardship of the year. I even went sledding with the kids! Since we were packing up to head back to Denver on Friday, we decided to have our Thanksgiving meal on Wednesday. So we all crammed ourselves into the relatively small kitchen and got down to business making our favorite recipes, while heavy snow fell outside the windows and the kids played happily. All in all, it was a really great day.

The way the vacation house was set up, our family of four was in two rooms on the basement level. It was quiet and cozy down there. I loved retreating downstairs to read, enjoy some quiet, pray, and email my new friend Kim. Thanksgiving morning, I woke up feeling a little more off than usual, but assumed it was from my fun-filled day of sledding and cooking and photographing the kids in the snow. As I swung my legs around to the floor and sat on the edge of the bed, I noticed my balance was way off. I was shaking.

I stumbled to the bathroom to see if I looked different. Sometimes I would wake up with Bell's palsy, which caused my face to droop on one side. Much to my surprise, I didn't have Bell's palsy, but something more unsettling. The muscle in my neck had collapsed overnight, causing my head to shake uncontrollably. Think bobblehead. I looked very much like a Parkinson's patient. Sure that it was a result of all the activities of the day before, I slipped right back into bed thinking, *It's fine; it will go away.*

Eventually, Forbes came down to our basement room to bring me coffee. When he cracked the door open, I sat up.

"Are you shaking?" he asked, worry in his voice.

"Yeah," I said, "I'm just really tired and cold from yesterday. I'll be up in a little bit."

Forbes went back upstairs, and I stayed in bed for a while.

Then I worried I was being antisocial, so I decided to climb the stairs to see everyone. I'd talked myself into believing that while I could feel the shaking, it wasn't that noticeable, so everything would be fine.

When I got to the second step, my sweet sister-in-law Katie called, "Good morning, Sis!" from the top of the stairs. When she looked down at me, her smile turned instantly to shock. *Well, I guess it is noticeable.* I'll never forget her face that day. A combination of total sadness and overwhelming concern.

Katie stood speechless as I stepped closer to her. When I reached her, she wrapped her hands around my shoulders and asked what was going on. I said I didn't know. She quickly drew me to a nearby bench to sit down, then went to get me a glass of water. As she got the water, Katie mentioned something about videoing my current state. I could hear her talking, but the rushing in my ears was louder than her words.

When she handed me the water, I shakily spilled it everywhere. Embarrassed and frustrated, I got mad and asked everyone to just let me be for a few minutes. They obliged. So I sat on the bench staring out the window, while everyone else tended to breakfast and the kids' needs.

In the next twenty-four hours, I worked hard to adapt to my new symptom. If I concentrated and held my head a certain way it wasn't as noticeable, so I decided to do that for the last days of our trip. By the time we returned home on Sunday I was beat, but my heart was full from having gone. Monday morning, I woke up with the shaking in full-fledged mode. Only now, I had no control over it.

At this point, I had Forbes on board with the Lyme theory. He was intrigued, supportive, and most important, prayerful. We began researching Lyme-literate doctors and Kim was busy doing the same. I'd read a lot about Lyme on our trip, even though I didn't discuss it with anyone, and had begun praying over possible protocols and doctors. One doctor Kim researched appeared to be the most experienced in my symptoms and, incredibly, was right around the corner from my family in Colorado. This meant I could stay with them if I could schedule an appointment.

I reached out to this doctor. To my surprise, he called me back himself and talked with me for fifteen minutes. Remember, this guy has no clue who I am, and I'm not his patient. He advised me to let the diagnostic center know about my newest symptom and if they ruled out Parkinson's, then I had something called neuro-Lyme. In that case, time was of the essence.

I needed help faster than immediately. Unfortunately, it was December, and the doctor was booked until August. Despite this, he told me to call him after I talked to the diagnostic center.

As requested, we sent a video of my latest symptom to the diagnostic center. This was immediately followed up with a phone call. Two days later, I had an appointment with the neurologist we had already seen in Atlanta.

We were fortunate to have family friends fly us to Atlanta. My recent decline made the four-hour car drive more than daunting. Forbes had a huge work deadline he was up against, so with my mom's promise to give him every detail and the ability to call in to the appointment if he wanted to, Forbes stayed home while my mom and I took the trip ourselves.

Once there, we met with the head neurologist at the center, my third or fourth encounter with him. During our first meeting, I didn't care for him at all. But with every appointment, I liked him more and more.

This appointment was different than the others. Instead

of being ushered into an exam room, we were taken to the neurologist's office, where we waited a good while before the doctor came in. He took a look at my new symptom and began to discuss Parkinson's with us at length. Afterward, he asked me to walk down the hall, away from him, without any help. My mom told him I couldn't do that. He asked me to "just try."

My mom stood next to the neurologist, while I turned my shaky, little weak self and mustered up the ability to walk down the hall, leg dragging and all. He looked at my mom and said, "She's really gone downhill fast in the last six weeks."

You can imagine the look on my mother's face. She would have loved to slap him at that moment. "Yep," was all she said with tears in her eyes.

I turned, using the wall for some assistance, then walked back into his office and dropped into a seat. Without hesitation, he said confidently, "You don't have Parkinson's, but something is definitely going on."

Oh, the comments in my head! After he rambled for a few minutes, it was my turn to speak. I asked what he knew about late-stage Lyme disease. He stared at me a long moment before answering. Finally, he admitted, "Not much, but it would explain almost all of your symptoms."

As we sat in his office, the neurologist called a colleague in the infectious disease department and said, "I have a patient in my office who I think has late-stage Lyme."

After what seemed to be a very long call, he hung up and spun his chair around to face us. He said he was really hoping their facility could help me so that he could watch me get better. Unfortunately, the other doctor said that because the lab results showed nothing, they couldn't do anything for me. He told me to keep my faith and not give up.

I had done enough research at this point to know that this was a possibility, so his answer didn't shock me. It gave me permission and validation to go down the path of finding a Lyme-literate medical doctor (LLMD). So the head-bobbing, my most alarming symptom to that point, became the biggest blessing. When we experience something extraordinarily hard, it's easy to assume God has left us. But sometimes God allows the unthinkable to happen so that we pursue Him to a depth we couldn't have known if we hadn't experienced that trial.

On the plane ride home, I stared out the window thinking over the past twenty-three months. We'd run an absolute marathon and now we were about to ski uphill. What was that going to look like? We had mountains ahead of us, but God gave me all the confidence I needed to take the next steps. We prayed hard that we would be in His will, that we would not move until He wanted us to. We prayed through the phone calls, the books, the reams of information. But I was determined not to move without God letting me know it was the move He wanted us to make.

I called the amazing doctor in Colorado back and told him that the neurologist had confirmed I didn't have Parkinson's. In light of that new information, he ordered specific blood work that needed to be done immediately. After researching, examining protocols, and praying for direction, we thought we found an LLMD on the East Coast. The doctor in Colorado knew of him, which was comforting, and said the blood work would jump-start the process for when I got an appointment. I had so many questions and so many hoops to jump through. It was amazing to see how, with every one that came up, God already had an answer and was preparing the way for me.

A sweet friend who worked at our local hospital and had

been on this journey with us from the start, offered to draw the samples needed. She then graciously mailed it to the lab.

I decided to get in touch with the LLMD who I believed the Lord was giving us peace about. We'd spent so much time praying and researching, and this seemed like the obvious next step. I called his office the second week of December and was told that he wasn't available until March. *Ummmmmm. What?*

Another wall.

Then the receptionist said that his partner could see me at the end of January. Even so, I was disappointed because, for some reason, I believed that this doctor was IT! Specifically, what we thought I needed was to follow his protocol.

Because Lyme is a somewhat puzzling disease to tackle, there are many different approaches to combating the disease. We felt strongly that the protocol this office offered would give me the highest potential to fight it. After I swallowed the lump in my throat, I asked, "Well, does she follow the same protocol as the other doctor?" The receptionist answered, "Absolutely. And once you're here, they'll work together with you." That was music to my ears.

"I'll take the late January appointment then!" I said. My excitement didn't change the immense pain or terrible symptoms I was having, but it gave me hope that we were finally on the right path.

{ *chapter eight* }

ALMOST THERE

Hope does not disappoint.

Romans 5:5 (NASB2020)

EVEN THOUGH THINGS WERE pretty rough, I tried to embrace every moment I could, finding joy in small things. I was starting to accept that I had no assurances about what the future held for me, so I needed to be part of everything I could. It wasn't that big of a goal, but it was something to shoot for.

Christmas season had arrived, which meant it was time for school parties. As much as I didn't want to go to the children's school and be stared at, I gritted my teeth and went. At the beginning of the school year, Elizabeth and I had signed up to help with the Christmas party. We even came up with a cute craft for the kids. Remember, at this stage of the game, I had zero coordination and my head was constantly shaking, so Elizabeth had me pass things out while she went around helping the kids glue things to their craft.

As I struggled to get the items needed for the craft out of a plastic bag, a little girl said, "Mrs. Sarah, do you have a tune in your head?"

I glanced at Elizabeth, confused. She shrugged.

"Baby, what are you talking about?" I asked.

She explained, "You know, a tune in your head," and started shaking her head back and forth like she was jamming to music. Tears filled my eyes and I looked back over at Elizabeth, then, with a smile, I told the girl, "I sure do have a tune, and it's a good one, too."

Oh my word, y'all, she thought I was just rocking out in my head! Little did she know, I had *no* control over my head or my neck.

I love children's innocent perspectives on things. That moment made me giggle and I felt, once again, God smiling down on me. He has a sense of humor, you know. It was a funny moment about a not-funny thing, and we just let it be funny. I walked away from the party thankful I went, despite how I looked, and thankful that a sweet-minded kiddo reminded me again that God was present in every moment, smiling down at His child.

Our Hail Mary

Christmas that year was full with wrapping up my photography business amidst joyful holiday celebrations with my family. We tried to soak in all the goodness and fun as much as possible. Unfortunately, my weak body had contracted bronchitis. So in addition to my other symptoms, I was really sick with barely enough energy to cough.

Christmas Day was literally a blur. I sat in front of the fire at my parents' house, passively watching life happen all around me. I had no words, no emotion, and no ability to engage at all. When it came time to gather around the dining room table, I stood by my chair to sit down. Suddenly, intense panic swept over me. Even though I'd learned to deal with the glaring changes my illness had caused, others hadn't. The thought of sitting at that long table with my constantly shaking head, barely able to lift food to my mouth seemed like more than I could handle. I discreetly asked my mom to move my place setting into the kitchen with the kids. She looked at me, confused. I explained that I just couldn't be on display one more minute.

"Mom," I said, "I can't even hold my fork. I just can't handle being watched right now."

There was a lot of pride in that statement, though I'm not sure how I had any left. But I did. Graciously, my mom picked up my plate and moved me into the kitchen, where I sat with the kids. After spending a minute or two desperately trying to use my fork, I decided to just sit and listen to the giggles of the children. It was much more enjoyable than fumbling with my silverware.

The day after Christmas, we all gathered again at my parents' house. My sister and her family were in town and the cousins were playing happily. I was wrapped in a blanket on the couch in my parents' den, absentmindedly listening to a conversation in when my phone rang. It was the LLMD's office in Maryland. An appointment opened up on December 28. Would I like it?

I could barely get my "Yes!" out fast enough. The woman on the phone said she'd email me the paperwork. If possible, she explained, I should send all my medical records and the forms that day. I can't count the number of pages of medical records I had at this point. By then, I was on my twenty-third month of being sick and had seen nineteen doctors! Due to my inability to hold a pen, my sister Mary printed out the twenty-something pages of medical forms and sat beside me, filling out every form. She then spent a significant amount of time sending the doctor's office all the necessary paperwork. The weather forecast for Maryland was a doozy, so we had to leave the next morning in order to arrive before the snow started. Thankfully, we were able to quickly arrange childcare for the kids with some dear friends.

Getting on that plane was probably the biggest leap of faith I'd ever taken, other than starting my business years before. The two may seem incomparable, but the feelings of vulnerability and hesitation were identical. I was getting on a plane to see a doctor for a possible diagnosis that might fit my symptoms—or at least that's what it looked like to everyone else. What we were actually doing was getting on a plane because God had ordered every single step leading to this moment. I got on that plane out of obedience and maybe just a bit of tenacity. Sometimes God asks us to do crazy things. A wise soul once told me that if you are a Christ-seeker, at some point God will call you to do things that don't make sense to other people.

In her book *Cultivate*, Lara Casey puts to words exactly what this next step felt like to me:

[A]s you step out in faith and continue along the path of following God, you will inevitably come to the point when you realize that, no matter what path He puts you on, the ultimate reward is a relationship with Him.[12]

At this point, I was a physical, shaky mess. Spiritually, however, my heart was thrilled about seeing how this next step would take me deeper into my faith.

Our plane arrived and we made our way to the hotel to rest up before my appointment the next morning. What do you do when you're super sick and it snows the entire day before your 8 a.m. appointment? You binge watch Netflix with your husband, of course! We felt so much intense emotion going into my upcoming appointment. Not only did we believe this was our Hail Mary, but also it was the first step down a very long road. So watching non-stop Netflix shows together was a welcome escape.

I would like to say that I woke up the next morning bright-eyed and bushy-tailed, but there was none of that left in me. What was left was the hope I had that Jesus led us here. Even if this didn't provide an answer, I knew we were supposed to walk obediently into this appointment. When we found the doctor's office, Forbes, my mom, and I quickly prayed together before walking in.

The office was nothing like I imagined it would be. It was a small and nondescript. As we went in, we were greeted by the incredibly kind staff. I'd already become fast friends on the phone with the girl handling all my paperwork, and she came out to give me a hug.

We then sat there for just a little while, until a very petite woman walked around the corner with the most calming, gentle smile I'd ever seen. She called my name and, with assistance, I stood up and walked to follow her. I felt the full range of emotions at this point. We went into the office and she asked me to sit on the table as another woman came in to assist her. My mom kept looking at me, and I kept looking at Forbes, all three of us trying to figure out which woman was the doctor. It took us almost ten minutes to realize that the woman who escorted us from the waiting room was *the* doctor we'd come so far to see. We had never in all of our experience of doctors' offices seen a doctor come out to get a patient. Although I researched Dr. S, I'd never seen a picture of her. Once we figured out that she was the actual doctor, we hung onto every word that came from her mouth.

Dr. S started with an assessment. She then had me walk down the hall, during which she walked beside me with that same calming smile, frequently reminding me, "It's okay." As I walked, my eyes welled up with tears. The weight of my emotions settled into this moment. Walking unassisted was hard and the self-sufficient pride left in me wanted to do it on my own, but the reality was that I couldn't.

Walking completed, we entered her personal office. Forbes and my mom held legal-size notepads, taking notes and asking questions. Dr. S began by asking my mom questions going all the way back to my childhood and then working forward. We were in her office a solid three hours. Interestingly, the longer we were with her the more confident we became in our decision to be here. She was patient, kind, caring, and incredibly knowledgeable. She was glad to share her knowledge with us and was remarkably encouraging.

Toward the end of the three hours, Dr. S told me what we had somewhat expected. She thought I had late-stage neuro-Lyme disease with several co-infections. *Co-what?* Co-infections, meaning I had several different types of bugs attacking my system at once. The doctor then went through each of them: bartonella, babesia, and borreliosis (Lyme). She explained what each bug was and how they affected—or rather infected—the body differently. She explained how some people with clinical symptoms of Lyme can also have white matter lesions on the brain. *Interesting!*

Dr. S advised me to remove gluten and dairy from my diet. The dairy, she explained, could be added back in later, but my gut issues were so severe that removing dairy would help give it a break.

At this, Forbes piped in. "Is there anything else she should remove? What about coffee and caffeine?" he asked. "Could that make things worse?"

If looks could kill, my husband would have died at that very moment, because my eyes shot daggers at him. She looked at him, then at me, and then back at him.

Finally, she said, "No, do not take coffee away. She won't be able to function without it."

HA! I thought. I know Forbes only had my best interest at heart, but coffee was my jam. With every other food that tasted good taken away . . . *do not mess with my coffee.*

Coffee issue settled, Forbes asked what we could do about my pain. I'd not yet confessed to Dr. S how bad it had gotten. Forbes proceeded to tell her that twice the week before, in the middle of the night, he found me on the floor in a ball rocking back and forth.

"Is there anything that could help with that?" he asked.

Then I was introduced to one of my loves I still cling to today: Epsom salt baths. I was so desperate to get better that I was willing to do anything Dr. S suggested. I even told her, "If you said licking a toad would make me better, I would do it." She laughed her sweet little laugh and said there would be no need to lick toads, but she was glad I was willing to follow the strict treatment plan.

Dr. S then went over what she suspected was the culprit, and began to discuss a treatment plan. She explained that after infections pass through the blood-brain barrier, IV antibiotics are recommended. I'd known about this before walking into the appointment because of the protocol we felt led to follow. However, once I heard her say it, I panicked. My uncle passed away two summers before from a staph infection in his PICC line, so we all cringed at the thought of me having one. Thankfully, Dr. S went over why that treatment is so effective, specifically in my case.

In case you aren't familiar with a PICC line, it's basically a long, thin tube inserted into the arm then threaded into the larger veins near the heart. Through that tube, antibiotics or other medication can be delivered directly into the body.

Dr. S explained that I would be monitored weekly with blood work and that a nurse back home would change my PICC line bandage. She also promised that this was the best course of treatment.

Looking at us all, Dr. S said, "Sarah has a very long road ahead of her, but she can do this."

She ordered many more tubes of blood. I'd kept track of how much of my blood had been drawn over the past twenty-three months. By this point, it had been over five hundred tubes. Dr. S would have some of the samples sent to different labs in different states, and it would take three to four weeks for results. Once she had the lab results, she could put everything together for a definitive diagnosis. Until then, she sent me home with lots of vitamins, oral antibiotics, herbs, and most importantly, hope.

If you're wondering why Lyme is such a puzzling disease or why it took me going further north to get answers, we did too. Typically in the Southeast, unless you have a rash from a tick bite and get tested quickly, you'll be hard pressed to find a doctor who will take it seriously or even know how to investigate. If we had lived in the Northeast, it likely wouldn't have taken twenty doctors to find a diagnosis.

After learning more from Dr. S, we did what most anyone would do. We asked how in the world I contracted Lyme? Had it been at work? I spent half of my days rolling around on the ground for photoshoots. Had it been on my most cherished trip, when Forbes and I went to Maine, where we hiked and mountain biked? We'll never know the answer, and that's okay. Regardless of *how* it happened, it happened. We were in this moment for a reason and simply had to push through.

Although we left Dr. S encouraged, we were heavy-hearted. It would take a lot for me to get better. We learned many more things about the disease that we hadn't known—how once it goes untreated for as long as mine had, there was no way to eradicate it completely. In other words, there was no actual cure.

So while I had hope of getting better, I didn't know what *better* would look like. I tried hard not to go there, because it wouldn't change anything. Dr. S promised she would work to get my immune system where it needed to be to, in a sense, suppress the infections.

As with every other doctor's appointment, Forbes, my mom, and I sat together afterwards to gather our thoughts and decide what to report to family and prayer warriors waiting at home. We had several friends fasting that day on our behalf, so we felt an urgency to report back. Forbes helped me write an email to those who needed to know. We didn't really have any answers or a direct diagnosis, but we had Dr. S's suspicions and the protocol we would follow if she was right. That was more than we had ever gotten before.

We came home with a slew of vitamins and herbs, and some antibiotics. Not long after, Mom and I headed to Target to get all the baskets and items needed to get fully organized. The next few days were spent processing the information we'd received, getting medicine baskets organized and notes written out, setting alarms on my phone for when to take my medicine, and buying healthy food.

We were trying to embrace this new normal, knowing that if Dr. S's diagnosis were correct, a new routine would begin. Incredibly, after only one week of my new daily regimen of forty-plus pills, my head stopped shaking! This confirmed that we were finally on the right track. But even with the excitement of the small progress I'd made, a lot of heaviness came with it.

For those who don't know, Lyme disease is one of the most controversial diseases out there. Coming back from my neurological appointment in December, I literally begged God to give me anything other than this disease. Because while I was fighting for my life, I knew I would also have to defend my every move with the naysayers around me. Each doctor and friend who'd never heard of Lyme and its treatment, who thought they knew better, would question each decision we made.

But this wasn't about them. It wasn't about Lyme disease either. The story God was writing was bigger than that, and I held on hard to what He was teaching me through each and every moment of this journey.

The Happiest and Saddest Day

A few weeks into the new year, I was doing the slightest bit better. While my head had stopped shaking, all my other symptoms mostly remained the same. However, I could sense a small difference in my hands' mobility that had me excited and hopeful.

On January 30, 2014, I received the phone call I'd been waiting on for two full years. While on my way for a massage, which I'd been getting weekly to help with pain, I pulled over in a parking lot to answer the call from Dr. S. I reached frantically for a scrap of paper, ready to write down every word she said.

My blood work was back, and the results made Dr. S both happy and sad. Her suspicions were correct. I had late-stage neuro-Lyme disease with two other co-infections as well as some other odd things in my blood, also caused by the disease. She gave me a lot of information all at once and, of course, added more supplements to my list. She then detailed the plan for next week. I was to begin IV antibiotics immediately, which meant she would get my paperwork together and line up my home healthcare to start the process. She would also send everything to my beloved Dr. B, so he could have all the information if anything came up locally.

I got off the phone and wondered, *Who do I call first? Forbes, of course!*

It was a little sad to be excited about being diagnosed with a terrible disease. But I was relieved. I had an answer after waiting and wondering for so long. I was finally able to give a name to what had been stealing my life from me for the last two years. I ran into the massage therapist's office shouting my news. My massage therapist hugged me, saying, "I'm so excited for you!" Then she stepped back and said, "I mean I'm so sorry that I'm excited. Is that bad?"

I was weepy, but answered with steely resolve. "No," I said, "I know what you mean. Now that I know what I'm dealing with, I'm ready and excited to fight this thing."

{ *chapter nine* }

SHOWING UP

Encourage each other and build each other up.

1 Thessalonians 5:11 (NLT)

BEFORE I GOT SICK, I was lucky enough to be a part of several groups of friends. I had friend groups from church, moms from the kids' school, and clients who had become like family. Honestly, I was kind of a social butterfly, and there was hardly a weekend evening when we didn't have plans to do something with someone. My faithful, introverted husband would just go with the flow, because he knew how much I loved people, that I never wanted to miss an opportunity to be with friends. I definitely had a serious case of FOMO (fear of missing out). I worked most weekends so there were many things I missed out on, but if I was available, we were there! Rain or shine! Tired or not!

During the week, I would have at least one girls' night with friends from all the different aspects of my life. Looking back on it now, I realize how busy I was. But being around friends energized me, and I loved hearing about their lives, having fun, and growing spiritually with them. The community I shared with these women helped fuel my creative side. It's a little hard to explain, but being surrounded by my people seemed to make me come alive.

Then, I got sick. Something had to give.

For those first few months, I was too prideful to admit to anyone, even close friends, that something was wrong. I was afraid people would look at me differently if they knew. I was afraid I would seem less reliable, weak, and less valuable. We live and learn, right? Looking back now, I wonder what could have been different if I had just been more honest. Would it have changed the outcome of many of my now-altered and even lost friendships?

As an Enneagram 9, my personality loves peacemaking and I'm always up for whatever makes others feel loved, because then I feel loved too. But there's a negative side to being an Enneagram 9. I avoid conflict and don't always know what I need. Knowing this helps make sense of how my unwillingness to admit something was really wrong created an issue within my friendships.

As the months dragged on, I became more honest with my friends about what was happening to me. But I still downplayed a lot of it because, again, I cared so much about what they would think about me. If they asked, I would just give a vague explanation like, "I've been having some random stuff going on and no one can figure it out." But then, as more months passed, dinner date invites slowed down. Weekends became time to rest and regroup for photoshoots. I started to feel like I was fading away both physically and socially.

As my symptoms increased and became more obvious,

most people had no idea how to react and so they just stayed away. For the record, I'm not sure if the roles had been reversed that I would have known what to do either.

Being sick or having anything out of the ordinary going on in your life is isolating in general. People aren't sure how to react because most people don't have a framework for responding to hard things. And when you sense that no one understands what you're going through, the loneliness can be overwhelming. For me, because my symptoms were multi-systemic with no explanation, it was uniquely more difficult for others to relate to me than if I had general diagnosis of a common disease. With a cancer diagnosis or a specific disease, there are typically a swarm of resources available. But for a long time there was nothing for me to point to that anyone could relate to or understand. So I found myself feeling isolated and alone.

As I got more and more sick, each day mimicked the day before, but in a slightly different way. It was like I lived in the movie *Groundhog Day*, but in this version, the main character gets worse rather than better. As if it wasn't hard enough to muster the energy to get up every morning and fulfill my duties as a mother and business owner, I began to experience something I couldn't have seen coming. The changes I saw happening in my friendships started to cause more hurt than the actual physical pain I was in.

I've always been an optimist and a fighter. The glass is always half full and when life gets tough, I get tougher. That's just until that tough exterior gets stripped away and takes my dignity with it. My glass half-full attitude was definitely on the verge of being knocked over and poured out. Fear was creeping in uncomfortably close.

One of the hardest things for me, and especially for

my extroverted personality, was that once I was really sick, I realized there was constant talk about me and my illness going on behind my back. It's never comfortable knowing you're the subject of conversations that you aren't a part of. Sometimes those conversations were out of concern for me, but often they were not.

I know that in a unique circumstance like this one, it made sense that people didn't know how to respond. They did the best they could. I'm sure it was hard and confusing for friends and acquaintances to watch the major changes happening to me. This wasn't something any of us had experienced before, and to be fair, it was still a mystery what was happening to me, a nameless affliction.

Wanting to be helpful, friends suggested a broad range of "solutions," from taking antidepressants to spending more time in prayer. I know they found it hard to believe that in our modern age of advanced medicine, I had no real diagnosis.

Without saying it, some friends felt that if the doctors couldn't figure it out, then maybe I was just mentally unstable. So while understandably trying to reclaim some normalcy, many simply drifted away. This was hard to experience, but what saddened me most was that those friends lost the opportunity to see God at work up close. I've learned the hard way that we can't see God working with our backs turned. And when we turn away, we won't know how to pray for our people. It's only when we sit in the thick of it with them that we experience that blessing.

Even though many of my friendships were altered during this dark time in my life, I had a handful of deep-diving women who were always right on time when I needed it most. I was also encouraged by many others. Clients I hadn't spoken to in a while would hear what was going on and text me encouraging words that meant the world. One client even dropped off a beautiful necklace and headband one day with a note that simply stated, *You are loved. Know that.* I felt it for sure. There were also friends I hadn't spoken to in a long time who graciously moved toward me, without knowing any details, to offer any help they could. And there were a handful of friends who boldly stepped into my life with humility and self-sacrifice to help carry the heavy burden of my illness.

There is a great picture of this type of friend in Exodus. It's a somewhat lengthy story, so I'll just give the gist here. While the Israelites were wandering around in the desert, the Amalekites attacked them where they were camping, a place called Rephidim. Moses told Joshua to "choose some of your men and go out to fight the Amalekites. Tomorrow I will stand on top of the hill with the staff of God in my hand" (Exodus 17:9). So as Joshua fought the Amalekites, Moses went to the top of the hill with Aaron and Hur following behind. As long as Moses held up his hands, the Israelites were winning, but when he lowered his hands, the Amalekites would beat them back. When Moses grew tired, Aaron and Hur brought a large stone so Moses could sit down. They even held his arms for him until the sun went down. *They held his arms for him, and the Lord brought victory for His people.*

While I was at my sickest, a friend came to my house three days a week, ten minutes out of her way, to pick up Warren and take him to school for me. Sometimes she would get to my house and Warren wasn't dressed. So she would dress him, too. I had other friends attend field trips with my kids for me. I had a friend offer to address Christmas cards because she knew sending cards was important to me. Friends would show up with food when we said we were fine because they knew we were definitely not fine.

When it comes to friendships, location is important, but it's not everything. Some of the dearest members of my support group lived more than four hours away. It's totally possible to ride out a journey with a close friend, even with miles separating you. While I was sick, phone calls and texts with my circle of friends kept me going.

In addition, people who didn't even know me were praying for me daily. Even now, occasionally I'll meet someone at church or with another friend who lights up when they hear my name and say, "I was praying for you when you were sick!" This humbles me to my knees every time.

This is how others, like Aaron and Hur, held up my arms when I couldn't. What I could not physically do, they did for me. When I didn't have the words to pray, they prayed on my behalf. When I couldn't speak because it hurt too badly to form words, they would sit next to me in silence so I wouldn't be alone.

One dear friend, while others in our circle and community questioned my sanity, resolved to support me despite her concerns. Her decision to stand by me was especially solidified after dropping by my house for coffee one morning.

She came into my kitchen that day and her heart nearly stopped. There I was, sitting at the counter, pale as a ghost, my hands bent like claws. Three fingers gripped my tea mug as my body shook back and forth. My ability to control my muscles almost completely shot. That friend told me later, that moment was when she knew she was in this with me no matter what.

She made a commitment in that moment to me and to our friendship, regardless of the circumstances or her understanding of those circumstances. And so, she kept coming. And she kept folding my laundry and helping with my kiddos. She kept listening and praying. And, her self-sacrificial friendship is part of the way God healed my heart while He was healing my body.

Sometimes we aren't sure if we should get involved in someone else's crisis. It's uncomfortable and awkward, maybe a little scary. But if you're a believer, you have the Holy Spirit, the Spirit of the living God in you. You can depend on Him for wisdom and discernment for how and when to enter into a suffering friend's life.

Oddly enough, the hardest moment came when I returned from Dr. S's office and was the closest I'd been to an answer since getting sick. For so long, no one could believe that none of my doctors could figure out what was wrong with me, and now that this functional doctor (read: pseudo-doctor for some) suggested I had something many perceived as a made-up disease, I knew I was in for it.

The fear of judgment that came with this new diagnosis sent me to my knees. I barely got the words of a desperate prayer out before a warmth came over my whole body, similar to the feeling almost eighteen months prior when I heard the Spirit whisper, *You are going to get better, but you're going to have to hold on tight.*

After that, it didn't matter at all what others thought or said. God was there. It was at that moment that I awkwardly, yet confidently, stood up in my bedroom and decided to put on the armor of God from Ephesians 6, not worrying for a second what others thought. It was a crazy feeling in light of my people-pleasing personality. That experience gave me confidence that could only come from the Lord.

The truth is, life doesn't stop when you have a crisis. Maybe it's a job lost, a marriage ended, a loved one's death, or a scary health diagnosis. All of these are life-changing events, but none of them can stop the world from happening around you.

It can feel like there are two layers to dealing with a crisis. The first layer is figuring out how to function with what you're going through. The second is figuring out how to avoid being mad, bitter, or sad that the world didn't stop for your issue.

I'll never forget an event speaker eloquently share her experience of having to run to the grocery store to pick up bread and milk just after hearing that her best friend's husband had been killed in the line of duty. She stood in the bread aisle shopping like things were totally normal, while in her heart she was shouting, *How can everyone be going about their business when our friend has just died?*

Galatians 5:6 says, "The only thing that counts is faith expressing itself through love." If there's someone in your life going through a tough time, be brave enough to sit with them. If you can't understand the struggle they're going through, ask God to show you how to understand. Ask Him to give you the compassion to make that person feel supported no matter what. Because the hard reality is that it's not about you. It doesn't matter if you can sympathize or understand or make sense of what's going on. It's about you *being there*.

Proverbs 17:17 says "a friend loves at all times." It doesn't say to love when we can relate or understand what the other person is going through. It turns out that God often reveals more of Himself to us and through us *because* we don't know what to do.

In my experience, the best way to be equipped to walk beside a loved one going through a trial is to rely on the Holy Spirit through prayer. When we rely on our own understanding, we miss out on witnessing the wonders of God. When we try to make sense of things that don't make sense, we rob ourselves and others from experiencing God in a way that words can't express.

So friends, sit and wait and pray. To the best of your ability, be quiet and listen.

For those in the middle of a tough journey, there may not even be enough words to describe your circumstances or your feelings about those circumstances. Be sure that prayer is the best weapon against whatever suffering is weighing you down.

I often wonder if I'd prayed more about being open and honest with my friends, whether that could have changed the trajectory of some of my broken relationships. I wonder, too, why I didn't share more openly what God was teaching me and how He was literally guiding every step I took. Would there have been less judgment and shame in the first six months of my sickness? Or perhaps after my diagnosis?

Fear is a liar. I can't help wondering if my unwillingness to be honest robbed many friends of seeing God up close and personal. Although I never lied about my circumstances, I let my pride and fear of being perceived negatively keep me from being totally honest about what was going on with me.

If you're suffering, I encourage you to let people into your story. It doesn't have to be a crowd of people, but it needs to be more than just one. When one part of the body suffers, we all suffer. And whether you're holding your friend's arms or letting them hold yours, being in it together can go a long way toward healing.

I've learned the hard way that real spiritual growth comes in broken places. Think crushed grapes becoming new wine. Let others travel with you on whatever journey you're on and give them the opportunity to be a part of God redeeming your story.

{ *chapter ten* }

STEPS TOWARD HEALING

Take one step at a time
Learning as you go
Life has many questions
So many things you want to know
One step at a time
The answers will become clear
Don't ponder on the questions
Just enjoy the time you are here.[13]

John F. Connor

THAT FIRST DAY OF finally knowing what was wrong felt surreal. The term *neuro-Lyme* quickly became familiar, its reality slowly sinking in as we spoke it again and again. We made phone calls the rest of that day, setting up my treatment plan and letting friends and family know what was happening. Once orders were put in for the PICC line, home healthcare had to be lined up and schedules set. It was a tedious process to say the least.

On February 4, I went to have my PICC line put in. The whole morning was kind of a blur, but I remember the doctor saying, "I heard you have a very difficult case and a fragile body, so they've called me down to put your PICC in."

Who called him and told him I was a difficult case? Was it the nearly $1 million of tests my body had endured that gave him this impression?

I laughed to myself, even in the soberness of the situation. I just said "Fine, let's get this over with."

Within ten minutes of having the line in, my body went into total shock. I couldn't breathe. I was terrified. I hadn't gotten worked up by much at this point, but this WORKED me up. I kept saying, "It really hurts and I feel like I can't breathe." But the nurse calmly told me, "Well, it's fine." Then she said, "Now, you'll just need to go have your first infusion before you leave the hospital." That didn't make me feel any better. On the inside I was screaming at the nurse, but I avoid conflict like it's my job, so I managed a nod and a weak smile as they rolled me out of the room.

Forbes and my mom helped me to the car for the short drive to the infusion center. I was still shaken up and in more pain than I'd already been in. Once we got there, a friendly nurse named Dana came into the room calling me *honey*, asking about my story, and getting warm compresses to help with the pain while she ran my very first dose of IV antibiotics. After an hour, I was feeling much better. I tolerated the meds well enough to go home. Unexpectedly, I became fast friends with Dana and wasn't quite ready to leave yet. Over the next few years, we became close friends and she was part of the story of healing and redemption God was weaving together for me.

While all this was happening, Forbes was in full-blown tax season and swamped with work. After getting back from

Maryland, we talked with my parents about what the next few months of treatment could look like. Forbes was concerned about helping me with my treatment and caring for the kids, while still keeping up with the demands of work. We discussed options, which included Forbes taking a six-month leave of absence to cover the amount of time Dr. S said it would take for me to get back on my feet. My parents were adamant that Forbes putting his work on hold was not an option. They insisted that he'd worked too hard to get to where he was in his career. With his permission, they would step in and make sure everyone was taken care of. So with that, my parents became my primary caregivers, along with my friend Elizabeth and others who helped with our kids.

The day after my PICC line placement, I started what would become my new normal for the next six months. My home healthcare nurse, Nurse Gwen was wonderful, which was a relief. You really get to know someone who comes to your house once a week for six months. She was yet another person I would have not known had I not gotten sick. As it is, she became like family.

My mom, Elizabeth, and Forbes were all there for the initial meeting with Nurse Gwen. My fine motor skills were still hindered by the effects of Lyme, so it would be a while before I could handle changing my medicine by myself. Gwen showed them how to change my medicine, flush the line, and all the other maintenance a PICC line requires. We started on a shared schedule so Mom wouldn't have to come in town every day to administer medication every day at mid-day. She and Elizabeth took turns doing the mid-day ones and Forbes handled the weekend ones.

On day two of the PICC line, Dr. S called to check on me. I

told her about my chest pain and asked if that was normal. She said it wasn't and ordered a chest x-ray to make sure the PICC line was placed properly.

Mom dropped me at my appointment for the x-ray, not thinking we would get an immediate result. A friend of ours happened to be the radiologist working that day. He'd seen loads of my scans, performed my spinal tap, and been supportive on the sidelines, curious about what was attacking my body. He came out to see me and said he was elated they'd finally figured out what was going on with me.

He then went on to say he reviewed my x-ray. "Your picc is about two inches closer to your heart than it should be. You need to have it fixed immediately."

HA! I knew something was wrong. I went in the next day to have the line pulled back to the correct location, but the nurse in charge didn't like the placement overall, so he replaced the whole thing. *OUCH!* But I immediately felt better.

The next four weeks had me finding a rhythm of supplements, infusions, and bandage changes. I'd been warned that things might get worse before they got better, and they definitely did. As the medicine killed the "bugs" inside my body, something called a *Jarisch-Herxheimer reaction* happened. This occurs when the "bugs" release toxins into the body that can exacerbate the symptoms. How do you get them out? Detox, detox, detox. I learned more about detox and its importance over that first month than I ever wanted to know. Making matters worse, the process made me feel sicker than I could have anticipated.

My friend Kim walked alongside me throughout my whole Lyme journey, but was especially educated about and helpful during detox. She taught me tricks to manage the side effects, some of which I was able to share with my doctor. The community of those affected by Lyme is one big circle of learning, encouraging, and moving forward together. There was real comfort in knowing I was part of a group of people helping each other beat back this disease.

At the end of every month I flew back to Maryland, accompanied by my mom during tax season, and then by Forbes once May arrived and the pressures of his job let up.

Dr. S monitored my blood work weekly but still needed to see me in person once a month. Every time we went to her office, we fell more in love with her and learned so much from her wealth of knowledge. Often, her partner would come in and talk to me during my in-office infusions. They had a great team approach, which we benefited from immensely. As soon as Dr. S thought I was ready, she would change my antibiotic and add more things in to boost my immune system. I would get a Meyers IV drip in her office, basically a vitamin cocktail, and then see her for around an hour at each appointment.

Afterward, Forbes and I would grab Chipotle for lunch and then fly home, all in one day. With each month, I was getting stronger and after about two and a half months, I could drive again. That newly regained freedom was exhilarating.

If I'm honest, treatment was incredibly hard. But the beauty of friendships through visits and lunch dates, meals brought by and playdates in my own backyard, glittered like diamonds in the midst of the darkness. During this time, it felt like God gently carved out this little nook in my life. There, quality time, fellowship, and visits seemed to last longer and have increasing depth. Friends would come by and I'd share little stories of how God had taught me something, how He was working a miracle through a new medicine, or how He provided an opportunity to share God's handiwork with medical staff. What an honor it always is to be able to share how God is working. I was thankful to have this extra, unhurried time with friends who graciously let me share how God was expanding my heart through this experience.

A few months into my treatment, both doctors felt I was ready for high-dosage vitamin C infusions. They'd given me articles to read, which explained how studies found that high doses of vitamin C could kill cancer cells. This led doctors to try it on Lyme patients as well. The vitamin C infusion was the only one I couldn't have at home. After what felt like a million phone calls, I found an infusion center willing to administer it.

Vitamin C sounds pretty innocent, doesn't it? It was by far the WORST infusion of them all. I got an infusion of it every other week, and it took me out each time.

The only good part about those appointments was that my sweet friend Katherine, who drew my blood samples in December, drove me to the infusion center and stayed with me for the two hours it took to get the infusion. When she offered, I asked if she was sure. It was a serious chunk of time to commit to. Her response was that she was totally sure and looked forward to sitting and chatting. I consider her to be one of my wisest friends, and I hang onto every word that comes out of her mouth, wondering what I'll learn next from her. She knew instinctively that this part of the journey was new and full of unknowns, and without hesitation, she signed up to be my infusion buddy.

That first day at the infusion center still stands out in my memory. Not really because the nurse butchered my arm and forgot to clamp the IV so I had blood ALL over my cute outfit. It stands out because having my friend sitting there with me for those two hours was significant. If I hadn't been going through what I was, we would have been too busy with our lives to stop and make time to say what was on our hearts.

Thankfully, I only needed five treatments of the vitamin C infusions and then it was over and deemed a success. Even after I was PICC-line free, I still needed immune support once a month. To make it easier, Katherine invited me to her house, where she administered my medicines in her kitchen for a year. The drip usually lasted an hour and a half and I was always overwhelmed by the effort she took to make sure I had everything I needed to feel comfortable and to keep me on the path of healing.

The Power of Two

If I was going the route of functional medicine, I was going to be all in. So while I knew Dr. S was doing everything she could to help me, I decided to bring in a new nutritionist.

A family friend, Uncle J, who's very knowledgeable about nutrition—especially supplements—met with me to discuss other supplements I may want to consider. He was amazed by and excited about the supplements I was already taking, but he suggested one additional protocol. Before agreeing to add it, I wanted Dr. S to "bless it" first. This friend's recommendation was that I take six *more* supplements in addition to the forty-three I was already taking. She took the time to read each label and talked with Forbes and me before deciding they were okay to add.

I started the second protocol and we added "Uncle J" to the mix of our monthly meetings. As elements of my treatment plan changed, he would adjust my nutritional supplements.

Every time we talked, he offered an encouraging word, told me he was praying for me, and always made me laugh. He was another godsend who was all in on the journey with me. And ultimately, he played a huge role in getting me to where I am now. Even today, I still take many of his supplements.

As each month of treatment rolled by, I gradually got better. With each new medication came side effects that were rough, but typically, after five or so days, they became manageable and often stopped completely. I stayed consistent with the detoxing and after a few months, I had the coordination to handle my own medicines. Nurse Gwen added an extension to my PICC line so that going forward, I could do everything regarding my medicine on my own. Because I was out and about more, I became pretty skilled at hiding my infusions. I once administered my meds in the rain on a soccer field, thanks to the rain jackets having great pockets. Even worshiping at church couldn't stop me. I sat in the balcony on Sundays so that halfway through the sermon I could start my medicine.

After six months, I had my PICC removed. After that, I stayed on oral antibiotics and supplements for another year. Slowly, I added exercise back in and began to ease my way back into life. Every step was intentional as I tried not to overdo it, while also not holding myself back. It was a weird stage to be in and it lasted about a year. But if I'm honest, I still struggle with this balance. It had been painful to be known as the "sick person," and I was *so* tired of it. When I finally started feeling like my energetic self again, I was eager to dive back into things. Working, volunteering, running! I was excited for people to look at me without pity in their eyes. When I think about it now, I realize that the pity I thought I saw was actually compassion.

I did look and feel better, but I also knew I had to be very careful not to relapse by doing too much, too fast. At first I was cautious, but as the months went on, I became less cautious and wound up paying for it. I'd get frustrated for a few days, regroup, and then start again. Kind of like sin struggles, right? We're aware of them, but somehow the busyness of life and demands of the world can mask them so that we wake up sometimes wondering, *How did that sneak up again? How did I let that happen?* It happened because of a lack of surrendering. So I have to come before the Lord, acknowledge my sin, and ask for forgiveness and the strength to not repeat it. When I rely on His Spirit for help with balancing life in this broken body I'm living in, I do so much better than when I run at my own unhealthy pace.

As hard as this process was for me, it was hard for others, too. The old Sarah was back as far as they could see, so I kept being asked for volunteer positions at church and the kids' school. For my health's sake, I had to pace myself with what I said *yes* to, which was tough for my never-say-*no* personality.

Four months after I had my PICC line out, I started having heart issues again. I was crushed. I'd been really rocking and rolling into my new routine of finding balance, so I was a little shocked at having problems again so soon. Honestly, I think I needed to be reminded early on that I wasn't invincible and that setbacks would likely be a continuous pattern in my life. They're just part of living in a broken body. Each time they happen, I'm reminded that God is sovereign. It may sound strange, but life is richer because of the setbacks and relapses. The truth is, being completely healed physically isn't nearly as valuable as being healed spiritually.

So, many cardiology appointments later, we made a new plan. Like that, a whole new regimen began. Short walks would lead to short runs, which gave me hope for getting back to some kind of normal.

Around the time of my latest heart flare-up, a dear friend called me. This is the same friend who introduced me to my husband, so anything she said had great merit to me. She told me about a family in which the father was struggling with vague neurological issues and asked if I might be able to reach out to them.

Fresh out of my own health crisis and knee-deep in a new routine of infusions, pain-relief massages, heart issues, and full-time caring for myself, I wasn't sure if I could help. But the Holy Spirit clearly said *yes*. So I reached out to Hannah, whose husband, David, was struggling with significant health issues.

We still laugh about how she thought I was a little crazy when I texted her, asking if I could meet with them to talk and pray. It felt completely normal to me at the time, so I know it had to be the Spirit. All I knew was that David was having neurological issues and that they were hoping I could connect him with the neurologist I'd seen at the diagnostic center.

However, before I got involved with their situation, I wanted to know how I could encourage and pray for them. Because I had *just* gone through something similar, I was full of what the Lord had taught me and also able to validate all the feelings and emotions this family was having. Looking back on it, I see now how odd it must have seemed that I felt so comfortable walking into that situation.

It actually worked out for me to visit them the next day. At the time, I looked a little bit like the Unabomber, with my heart monitor strapped to my chest and wires hanging here and there. But they didn't see that side of me. I dressed to hide the wires, because, after all, I was the "crazy lady" asking out of nowhere if I could come pray with them. I felt the need to look extra presentable.

At their home, I discovered a dismal situation. It had been an overwhelming blow for a young, successful father of four to be completely taken out by illness. David had this crazy symptom that made his head snap back and forth, which was different than the bobblehead I'd had. There was a name for this and it sounded legit, so I never entertained the thought that his situation could be anything like mine.

For hours, I sat and listened and cried and prayed with them. I shared my story, not because I thought David had Lyme, but because I wanted to communicate that I understood all too well how it felt to have more questions and symptoms than answers. They seemed thankful for the time I spent with them and for the encouragement. Because I had a full afternoon ahead, I promised to reach out to my neurologist the next morning. I hugged each of them and left with a pit in my stomach. It was as though I was reliving all the emotions of my story with them.

I'd been with them so long that I forgot to pick up my son and Elizabeth's son from school that day. I'd had zero cell service, so I missed all the phone calls from the school wondering where I was. Luckily, it was a small school and they knew there must be a good reason why I wasn't there, so they gave our boys cookies and snacks and let them play in the office. For the record, I was only thirty minutes late. When I finally arrived, I was mortified, but the boys were having the time of their lives. I explained a bit about where I'd been and the teachers were gracious and compassionate about the situation. They understood, having just gone through all of this with our family.

Before I could email the neurologist about David's situation the next morning, I received a phone call from his wife, Hannah. She told me how they'd stayed up all night praying and felt like they should go see Dr. S in Maryland. "Can you help us with this?" she asked.

I was a little taken aback by the rapid development, but told them I'd be happy to put them in touch with her. I was elated they'd chosen my doctor, but also a little surprised since just a few days before they had specifically wanted to see my neurologist. I had full confidence that whatever David had, Dr. S could figure it out. Even with that confidence, I wanted them to choose her, not me.

When I got home, I emailed Dr. S. She immediately responded with instructions for what David needed to do until she could get him an appointment. Within a week, he had an appointment, and off they went. I anxiously awaited their phone call about Dr. S's thoughts. Unbelievably, David ended up having the very same thing I had. *Say what?!?* The disease just affected his muscles and body differently than mine. When his symptoms began, someone gave him a steroid shot, which exacerbated everything. Treating Lyme with steroids is like pouring gasoline on fire. So what took two years to come to full fruition in me, took him only months.

David started on the same protocol I'd been on and we entered into his Lyme journey together. He'll tell you now that there were a few times he wished I hadn't gotten involved. Mama Bear came out every now and then when David needed some motivation to continue treatment. However, Hannah and I could only fight so much for him. David had to want to fight too. But with some firm reminding, he stayed on track.

It was a gift to share all I had just learned on my own journey with Lyme. I was so grateful for all the things Dr. S, my friend

Kim, other friends, and the good Lord had taught me. As with most treatments, things got worse before they got better, but over the course of a few months, David improved. He ended up with his PICC line being placed in almost ten months. He had even more undoing to do than I did!

I share that story only to show how one hard situation ended up helping someone else get solutions to their hard situation much quicker. But I had to be willing and available to offer what I had when it was needed. Even though it was completely out of my comfort zone, I'm thankful the Holy Spirit prompted me to help this family and grateful that I didn't miss it.

I believe God allows us to go through difficult things to teach us more about Him, but also so that we can help others in similar hard seasons. Ultimately, what was most remarkable was how our similarities in suffering created a bond between our families that has continued into the present. There is a depth to our relationship with Hannah and David's family that words will never really be able to describe. Looking back, I see how God brought me to them just like He'd brought Kim to me.

In a related way, this sort of deep connection is what Dr. S and I share. Through the journey of my illness, Dr. S became a dear friend to me. Real vulnerability and healing have taken place over the years we've known each other, and a cherished friendship is the result. Through David and I sharing our stories and experiences with others, there have been opportunities for Dr. S to help people we know and others in our community find physical healing through her methods. It's incredible to see how God is still writing this story.

Our stories started a small buzz around town and the surrounding cities. As a result, I ended up speaking at our church about what the Lord had taught me over the two years I was sick. Those who heard me talk that night shared my story with other families. Before I knew it, I was getting multiple calls throughout the week asking for help. It became so intense that I would ask people to text me first. Then I would schedule a call with them, as each phone call usually lasted several hours. I wanted to be able to give my undivided attention to each phone call because every story was unique, with some being more intense than others. Some of those who were newly diagnosed were terrified by my story, but I assured them that quick diagnosis was key and that they would be fine in due time. When cases go untreated for a long time is when things become more complicated.

As time passed and I adjusted to saying the right *yes* and the right *no*, I tried to figure out if and when to start working again. We were ready to get our lives back and wanted to do all the things we hadn't been able to for so long. One of those things was moving into a different home. So after ten years of being in the same house, we moved into a new one.

It was like we were given a fresh start. I kept telling friends that I felt like God was offering me a do-over. My prayer was that this time around, my life wouldn't be defined by constant busyness and personal pride but by an intentional and genuine pursuit of His purpose and plan for me. I was determined that the people He gave me to love and do life with would *always* be top priority.

{ chapter eleven }

GROWTH THROUGH TRIALS

We can ignore even pleasure.
But pain insists upon being attended to.
God whispers to us in our pleasures,
speaks in our conscience,
but shouts in our pains:
it is his megaphone to rouse a deaf world.[14]

C.S. Lewis

FRIENDS, THE BIBLE PROMISES us that we'll experience hard things in life. There's just no way around them. Some hardships we're born with and must learn to accept, while others seem to come out of nowhere, knocking the breath out of us. The important thing about difficult seasons is what you do with them.

Joshua 1:9 encourages us to "[b]e strong and courageous; do not be frightened or dismayed, for the Lord your God is with you wherever you go" (ESV). God wants us to have a faith strong enough to withstand the storms of life so that we don't just come out battered, bruised, and limping, but that we walk out upright, better, stronger, knowing Him more deeply.

A sermon by Levi Lusko, pastor of Fresh Life Church, resonated with me as it outlined what it means to be *anti-fragile*: "When life hits you hard, you actually get stronger. A wind extinguishes a candle, but fuels a fire."[15]

My hope is that after a hard season, I can say with hope these words from Lusko's sermon:

"I'm better because of it. I would never have picked to go through it, but because God allowed it, I faced it with worship . . . And on the other side of it I'm actually better, I'm actually faster, I know more of God's grace, He has revealed Himself to me in the midst of the fiery trial."

Whatever you're walking through right now, let it be used for His glory as you cling tight to God's promises through a difficult time. Let the struggle fuel the fire within you. Don't give up on God, even if it *feels* like He's given up on you. I promise He's there in the midst of that storm.

Just to be clear, I don't think I'm an exceptional Christian giving you "holy" advice on how to live your life. I'm just a normal human who walked through a really dark time and, in the midst of that darkness, saw God in a completely different way. I genuinely feel blessed to have gone through that hard season so that I could encounter how real God is and experience deep spiritual growth because of it.

Going on, Lusko said "[i]t is an incredible honor to be trusted with pain." Even though I wouldn't have asked for it, the gift of walking through a difficult time in order to meet God in a deeply personal way and see Him as more real than I imagined—that's something I wouldn't trade for anything.

Steven Furtick, pastor of Elevation Church, explained in a sermon titled "Ghosted," how "in the absence of answers, faith is born."[16] I've been trying my hardest to express this exact truth to you throughout this book. For me, the power of God's presence became real during this journey He took me on. I felt it through my core the entire time I was sick. I felt His presence so strongly at times that I ached for those around me to know just how real and near God was.

I started calling these my "stand-on-a-table" moments. Not in a table-dancing way (that would be insanely inappropriate), but in a "if-I-stand-on-the-table-and-shout-you-might-actually-pay-attention-to-what-I'm-saying-about-this" way. Kind of my version of "shout it from the rooftops."

I have a lot of moments during which I want to stand on the table or shout from the rooftops but, no, I don't actually stand on the table or climb onto my roof. I just want so badly for my children and my family and my friends and *you* to know how real and how near God is. Through my darkest of dark days, I felt His presence more than I felt alone. The feeling was, and still is, indescribable. Ultimately, it changed my life.

If God had given me the answers I wanted just months into my journey, or even after a year, I would have missed out on so much growth. Through the pain, the suffering, the sleepless nights, and the mystery, a faith emerged that I never knew possible. So much so that I would be remiss not to share it with anyone who will sit with me longer than ten minutes. I don't by any means love admitting that I'm a sick person stuck in a sick person's body, but I do love talking about how amazing our God is, how He is in every detail of every redemptive story. Even those stories that go on for years and years. Every moment has purpose for what lies ahead.

As my faith has deepened through this journey, I've also learned about being intentional with every decision, experience, and relationship.

Just this morning, years after my illness began, I was reminded of how vital it is that I pay attention to what God is revealing to me through His Word and His creation and the people in my life. While on a run today, I ended up on my parents' dock, just down the street from our home. Though concentrating on getting my best mile time in, I noticed splashing out of the corner of my eye. I stopped and stood still for a moment, looking down.

The tide was low but still coming in, and there in the marsh was a beached dolphin struggling to get back to the water. Frantically, I called Forbes. He was getting ready for the day, but I didn't care. I told him to get down there and help me rescue this dolphin! As I waited for Forbes, I devised our dramatic dolphin rescue. Just then, the dolphin began rocking back and forth until it got unstuck from the mud and headed to the water.

What a relief! Forbes was off the hook and I didn't have to stress about whether this dolphin would make it or not. But afterward, I couldn't help but consider how that dolphin's determination to get back where he belonged felt relevant to my life.

Am I being intentional about being where God wants me? Am I making the effort to pay attention to what He's revealing to me? Am I staying the course He's set out for me? Or am I just floating along, letting myself get stuck in the mud of my circumstances because I'm not actively paying attention or pursuing Him?

Years later, He's still bringing me back to that truth, a truth I'm meant to be living in.

Recently, a dear friend shared yet anot
that was spot on for what I know now. I
"I See It Now," Dharius Daniels referen
when he says, "Just because something
now doesn't mean it doesn't make sense
experiences and the tragedies that befell him, Daniels reflects
on how Job remained faithful and in the end, God revealed
Himself to Job and blessed his life.

Similar to Job, Daniels described how each of us can
discover that "the thing [you] thought was destroying [you] is
the thing God used to develop [you]." My illness has been the
thing God has used to create a living, breathing, undeniably real
faith in me.

After chapters and chapters of essentially debating with
God, Job repents and confesses: "My ears had heard of you,
but now my eyes have seen you" (42:5).

If anything can sum up the story of my illness and my faith
being made new, it's that verse. I knew all the Sunday school
answers, had my quiet times, prayed before meals, went to
church, and thought all of that was what real faith looked like.
Then that hard thing came around the corner and knocked me
to the ground. After walking through the fire, the valley, and
the storm, I can now say that I have *seen* God. I have seen His
hand on my life and I see His creation and I see His heart for
me every time I open His Word.

And so, here I am, fully believing that God had a purpose in
leading me through a season of illness. To quote another sermon
from Steven Furtick, "God has gifted me with my experiences
to fulfill my purpose and to build His kingdom."[18] Similarly,
Jennie Lusko says in *Fight to Flourish*, "There's a purpose in our
pain: to speak and sing of who He is and not be silent."

n't want to be silent about what He's done in me and for hrough the pain I experienced. I want to stand on all the bles and shout it from all the rooftops.

It was a long road that got me to this place. Yours may be a long road, too. I'd like to tell you that at the end of that road is complete healing in this world, but I can't do that. I wish I could say that if God had healed me completely, I would have still been faithful. But I'm pretty sure I wouldn't have been. What I can unreservedly tell you is that not being completely healed physically is God's grace for me, His "severe mercy"[19] that has made my life more full and more beautiful than a perfectly healthy body could ever have done.

My prayer and hope for you is that when you aren't getting the answers you want, when the burden you've been entrusted with feels too heavy to carry, that you'll remember that God is in the business of healing souls, not just bodies. His promises are real. Despite His ways being so much higher than ours that we can't comprehend them, they are always, *always*, better. And, sometimes it's only through broken bodies, broken homes, or broken hearts that He can fully heal our souls.

Ultimately, whether in this life or the next, when God has calmed the storm and cleared the way and made all the wrong things right, *you will see.*

Part 2

SEEING GOD THROUGH IT ALL

{ *chapter twelve* }

BEAUTY OUT OF MESS

Yet, God has made everything beautiful for its own time.
He has planted eternity in the human heart,
but even so, people cannot see the whole scope
of God's work from beginning to end.

Ecclesiastes 3:11 (NLT)

AFTER OUR SECOND BABY was born in 2010, we realized it was unlikely we'd have another child biologically. My pregnancy with Warren had been hard, and it didn't feel wise to do that again. So adoption became a topic of conversation between Forbes and I in the event we decided to add a third child to our family.

Years later, even after I was sick, we continued to talk about the possibility of adopting one day. We knew we wanted to, but just weren't sure about the timing. We struggled with all the usual adoption concerns, and obviously my health was a significant factor. The possibility of future relapses or flare-ups was very real, leaving us apprehensive about making long-term plans. While I'd been physically present with my children from 2012 to 2014, I was often mentally and emotionally absent. I'd also spent a great deal of time away from my family at doctors' offices or traveling to clinics, missing out on so many joys of motherhood. All of this had to be taken into account as we considered adding another child to our family.

At the beginning of my illness, we looked at orphanages online assuming that whatever was going on with me would be short lived. Once I was finally better, we weren't sure if we had missed our window of opportunity, and we certainly weren't getting any younger. Months would go by and when Forbes would bring it up again, I would still be undecided. More months would go by and I would bring it up. Then he would be undecided.

In the fall of 2015, at ages 35 and 36, we were still settling into our new home and our new normal. Right about the moment we were feeling content, God started tugging on both our hearts at the same time. We knew it was time to get serious about adoption.

I'm a firm believer that God won't call one of us to something that isn't meant for both of us. As we started to talk about it and pray, we knew every person in our lives would think we were insane. Eighteen months prior, I had a PICC line in my arm, was diagnosed with an essentially incurable disease, and was nearly at death's door. So we kept the possibility of adoption on the down low, until we felt sure. Really sure. One way to be sure something is worth pursuing is when all the *what-ifs* don't come to mind at all. When you stop at *I know God is calling me to do this* and all the fear stops at that sentence.

And yet, we didn't know where or how to start. So we started with prayer. Then we made lots of phone calls. My sister

Mary had adopted her sweet Hannah three years prior, so she was our greatest resource and support team member. She knew that adoption had always weighed heavily on our hearts, so she was one of the few we handpicked to join us on this adventure before we let others in on it. We were also fortunate to have a local ministry called Love One nearby. Love One supports families through the adoption process, offering resources for adoption, foster, and orphan care. They host a dinner once a year with a speaker, local resources, and agency representation. It was at one of these dinners when we were encouraged that the process might not be as overwhelming as we once thought. We walked away from that event with our hearts fully set on giving a child a loving home.

Forbes always believed that his strong desire to adopt a child from a Spanish-speaking country was from the Lord. I think he envisioned bringing home a little four-year-old boy we could love and adore. He would learn to play soccer, which would already be in his bones, and we would have another little soccer player in the family. My desire to adopt came without strong feelings of ethnicity or gender. I just wanted to adopt internationally. Really, I wanted to be obedient and bring a child who needed a family into ours. Because of Forbes's hope for a Hispanic child, we pursued it. I started calling Christian international adoption agencies, asking a ton of questions.

Much like my health journey, every call I made was just one step closer to the child the Lord was leading us to. A few weeks into pursuing the international route, through some wise words from an adoption agency, God closed the door to international adoption. At that time, the countries we were feeling led to adopt from all required staying in-country for up to five months before we could bring a child home. The burden that would have placed on our two children and our family as a whole made that an option we couldn't consider. A few other countries we were interested in weren't allowing international adoptions at all.

This is probably the part of the story where you expect us to be sad and confused. But we weren't. We'd walked into this journey, daily praying the words from James 1:5: "If any of you lacks wisdom, you should ask God, who gives generously to all without finding fault, and it will be given to you." When God closed the doors to international adoption, we knew that was His guidance and wisdom.

Once international adoption was removed from our growing list of options, we focused on domestic adoption. Obviously, with that decision, there was a new, even longer, list of questions. Would we adopt through foster care or a private agency? What age child were we willing to take? Were we interested in an open or closed adoption? On they went.

We dove right into every question, seeking Christ and answers. We went to a beginners' class through the Georgia Division of Family and Children Services (DFCS) in our hometown to learn more about foster care. We made phone calls to private adoption lawyers, met with our pastor, called agencies galore. I knew several people who had adopted through the foster care system, so I felt like that route could be for us.

So we filled out the appropriate paperwork. Then I headed to DFCS to turn it in and to find out when the next weekend class for foster parent accreditation would be held. A social worker came downstairs, sat on the bench with me, and told me how long the wait might be for a foster-to-adopt situation. She explained that we might have ten placements in our home before we had a child eligible for adoption. She wasn't very encouraging, but my tendency to be overly optimistic had me thinking, *Well, that's not going to be us!*

The very next day a private adoption lawyer, who had previously worked for DFCS, spoke some truth to me. She shed light on the reality of foster care. She also knew my health history and asked me a number of helpful questions.

"Sarah, do you think your children could handle having up to ten placements before you have a child you could adopt? They've been through so much in the past few years. Is this really something you want them to endure?"

Boom!

After that, I couldn't hear anything else she said. I just heard the rushing sound of my heartbeat in my ears. She crushed my dream with one question.

Even though our children were young when I was sick, Audrey had been very aware of what was happening. Over a two-year period, she saw her very active mom deteriorate to a shell of a human. At times, her tender heart could barely process it all. We tried so hard for things to feel normal, and as much as I'd like to say that it didn't affect her, Audrey was very affected by my illness and the aftermath. We had to consider this and her healing process as we thought through adoption options.

For the next week, we prayed constantly. We met with godly people, asking for help to make sense of it all. How could this not be for us? There was a need—a need we could fill!

After much prayer and a lot of heartache, we decided fostering-to-adopt was yet another door closed for us. We were one step closer to finding out what we were supposed to do, but I was sad because I'd been so sure that path to adoption was for us. There were so many children in the foster care program.

How could God tell us *no*? As the weeks went by, it became even more clear that it just wasn't the option for us.

Now what? Private adoption agencies? Really?

Still struggling to get over the overwhelming need for foster-to-adopt families, we began to look into domestic agencies. At this point, the two things that we *thought* we should pursue had been essentially closed to us. Even though it stung, I knew it was God leading us along the path He had for us.

As Forbes and I mulled over all those things, we were still unsure what age child we were to adopt. But we did know one thing: we didn't want to adopt an infant. We'd done the infant thing twice, got the t-shirt, and gratefully moved on. More than that, we knew that there were so many other families who couldn't have a biological child and wanted the experience of having an infant.

That fall, the Lord placed a distinct burden on my heart, along with the hearts of a few ladies at our church, for a women's retreat. Unexpectedly, I found myself taking the lead. In addition to all the thoughts of adoption and questions of what to do, I suddenly had to choose an event speaker. I needed to clear my head. I needed to go on a run.

I ran down to the community dock in my neighborhood and sat down to catch my breath. It was a beautiful day and I was thankful to be outside. I sat listening to podcasts of the speaker we ended up choosing. As I sat there, concentrating on her words, I had the strangest feeling I've ever experienced. There was a gentle urging to keep looking up, almost as if an invisible hand was lifting my chin.

I looked up from my phone for a split second again and again. Then I stopped and really took a look. Above me in the sky was a pod of pelicans.

"Those birds You created sure are pretty. Thanks for showing them to me," I told God a little insincerely. But I kept watching them. Then chills ran down my spine. God was trying to tell me something. You know the feeling. It's unshakable.

I sat a little longer, taking in the lovely view. And then I got up and ran back home.

As I got closer to my house, I couldn't get the pelican experience out of my head. *Why would God show me pelicans? I mean, I've seen them my whole life. Undeniably, they're cool birds, but what was He specifically trying to show me?*

I was still puzzled when I got home, so I pulled out my laptop. I typed into the search engine, *Christian symbolism of pelicans*. Yes, it sounds insane, but I needed to know why on this particular day God wanted me to notice pelicans. Several images popped up, but the one that stood out most was a mama pelican, her wings open wide, with three baby pelicans underneath her.

A Wikipedia article that featured the image said,

[I]n medieval Europe, the pelican was thought to be particularly attentive to her young, to the point of providing her own blood by wounding her own breast when no other food was available. As a result, the pelican became a symbol of the Passion of Jesus and of the Eucharist since about the 12th century.[20]

Other websites stated that the pelican was a symbol of sacrifice. I chewed on that all day until Forbes came home.

The dock experience was an odd one that I couldn't shake. I mulled over what it could mean. I prayed, asking for wisdom. I knew God was calling us to make more of a sacrifice. The call to adopt was not about us, but about the child He wanted to place in our home. Remember how we said we didn't want an infant? Well, now our question became, *Does He?*

We spent the next few months praying, researching, and making many more phone calls. We looked several times into working with a Christian consulting company that helps families through domestic newborn adoption. Twice in a three-month period we printed out all the information and went to sign on the dotted line, but couldn't do it. We still weren't sure that an infant was what He wanted for us. By then, we'd discussed it all so much that our heads were spinning.

While attending our church's Christmas Eve service that December, I pondered what had transpired over the last year and wondered what was to come. We were still in the thick of determining the adoption route the Lord wanted us to take. Unexpectedly, I found myself smiling as I began to cautiously hope that at next year's Christmas Eve service, I would have a child in my arms.

Finally, in January, Forbes suggested we go a week without talking about adoption. We had talked enough. He wanted us to each pray, to seek and listen on our own. Then we'd go to dinner that Saturday to talk about how the Lord had spoken to us.

My mind raced with all kinds of information. I felt we kept taking steps forward and backward, but still remaining unsure. Tuesday morning that week, I poured my heart out to my sister, then said I was going on a run because I thought it might clear my head.

I started out with the anticipation of running through my neighborhood. I ended up on my parents' dock to pray. There was a place on their dock that felt like "my spot." It's where I went when I really needed clarity.

I was only a few minutes into my run when I started having the same strange feeling I'd had on the dock back in October. Only this time, I felt that my whole person was being pulled toward something. It was like a gravitational pull to my prayer spot.

Well, okay then. I guess I'm bagging my run and prayer it is then!

As I approached my spot on the dock, I saw what appeared to be a palm branch from the night before. A storm had come through, so I figured it had washed up on the floating dock. But, as I got closer, I realized it wasn't a palm branch. It was a dead pelican—in the same spot where I normally sat and prayed.

I walked closer to it, then stood over it with tears streaming down my face. My thoughts rushed through my brain like a speeding train that wouldn't stop. I couldn't believe that God had sent me a sign. But . . . *What does this mean?* I texted my sister because I had no words. The tears kept streaming.

I moved my prayer spot to a different place that day. Sometimes, we have to approach something from a different angle in prayer. I'd kept praying the same thing over and over, but this day God showed me that I needed to change direction.

Feeling baffled, shaken, honored, and humbled, I went home. I made a few phone calls to Elizabeth and to another dear friend from church and told them what happened. The whole experience was too bizarre to share with many people. So I called a spiritual leader in my life and asked if she and her husband could meet me for lunch the next day.

When we sat down, there were knots in my stomach and I had zero appetite. I told them I wanted to meet because I knew they would give me godly advice, not just their opinions. I wanted help deciphering what this experience meant, though I knew they might not have immediate answers. After all, they had no idea what I was going to tell them. I explained that I wanted them to have all the facts so they could pray and hopefully help.

I started with the story dating back to October and finished with the dead pelican incident the day prior. I showed them a photo I'd taken of the dead pelican. And yes, I took a photo. It was too surreal not to! I explained that I wasn't sure if this meant I needed to stop pursuing adoption or to keep forging ahead. Did this mean God wanted even more of a sacrifice than we were willing to make? What *did* this mean?

They both smiled, which I think had to do with their love for how God speaks to us when we're paying attention. I could have totally missed this experience if I hadn't been actively seeking and anticipating His answer to our prayers.

I wonder how many times we miss God speaking to us because we throw up a prayer like it's an item on our to-do list. And then, if someone asks if we've been praying about it we can say *yes!* But, how many of us are truly looking for and expecting God to speak to us through signs, circumstances, and Christ-seeking people? He's not going to leave us all dead pelicans, but if we're paying attention, we *will see* His unmistakable hand in the circumstances around us.

Forbes and I were still in the middle of that week when we'd promised not to talk about adoption with each other, which made this much harder. Despite my high state of emotion, I honored that promise. But it was tough! Which is why I had to talk to this couple. I needed to get it all out. They encouraged me, prayed with me, and said they strongly felt God was not telling us to stop. He was encouraging us to keep seeking Him and pursuing His will.

Saturday came, and I couldn't wait to finally talk adoption

that night. Of course, Forbes's idea of a date is dinner and a movie. Yep, I had to sit through an *entire* movie before I could tell him anything. An agonizing two and a half hours later, we finally sat down at the restaurant.

I excitedly told him the story about my run and then leaned forward to show him the photo of the dead pelican on my phone. My words would not have done the story justice. He was speechless for a few minutes. Remembering that pelicans symbolized sacrifice and death to self, Forbes was struck by the image and what it meant for us.

His eyes filled up to the brim before an actual tear came down his face. He shared that after the last week of prayer and considering what God seemed to be revealing to us now, he felt we should adopt an infant domestically. It was not at all where we'd started, but we wholeheartedly believed it was where God had led us. Adopting an infant was going to be a huge sacrifice, not only for us as we were in our mid-thirties, but for our whole family. We were all in this together, though, and when God speaks, we move. Isn't it just like God to give us exactly the opposite of what we *thought* we wanted.

Utter excitement and peace took over our week as we placed calls to our friend, Donna, who worked with Love One, the local adoption ministry. She had joined us on our adoption journey months prior and was thrilled that we had peace about our decision. At that time, Donna wasn't able to write our home study, a requirement for adoptive families, so she advised us to use a local agency. Much to my surprise, the woman tasked with doing our home study was Mrs. Barton, someone I'd known growing up.

Mrs. Barton's children were my sister's age, and we'd known their family for years. That took a weight off and also made the process comfortable and enjoyable. We made it our goal to have our home study finished by the end of tax season in late April, which gave us roughly four months. Forbes' job would have calmed down by then and we felt that was a good goal for us. I was working very little, so I made it my full-time job to meet our home study goal.

There was loads of paperwork in addition to the four home visits we would have before we could officially apply to adopt. I made appointments, ran errands, went to the health department, the police station, etc. I would tell Forbes where to meet me during lunch breaks for fingerprinting and other requirements we needed him present for. I also scheduled a photo shoot with one of my friends so I could get cracking on our profile book.

Mrs. Barton met with us several times in our home and with our kids. The meeting with our children was a fun one. It was adorable to hear the kids' excitement about adding a sibling to our family. They said the cutest things, and I really wished I'd recorded that meeting!

I worked intently on designing and writing our profile book and on my birthday, one week before tax season was over, everything was complete. Books were ordered and ready to go, and so were we! As much work as we had done getting everything completed to apply to adopt, we still felt a good bit of apprehension. The paperwork was something we could do. It was the physical part of the process that we could check off the list. But we knew there was so much more to preparing for this next step than just paperwork.

The moment we'd felt the tug on our hearts to adopt, Forbes and I made a daily commitment to seek the Lord and pray together. We started getting up an hour earlier than normal and pored over books, online adoption resources, devotionals, and online sermons to prepare for what we were about to take on. We wanted to be as prepared as we could possibly be.

After a great deal of prayer and a multitude of phone calls, we decided to work with an in-state private adoption company. We mailed the box of home studies and profile books and then the waiting began!

At first, it felt so good to have finished everything up that I reveled in finishing such a huge project. As the months went by, however, the waiting got harder . . . and harder. As we waited and continued on with our regular everyday life, Forbes and I consistently sought Christ for guidance. The kids prayed at night. Forbes and I prayed every day throughout the day. Through it all, the craziest, most beautiful thing was happening. I was falling wholeheartedly in love with a child that I hadn't met. I had no clue if this child was a girl or a boy. I had no idea where he or she would be born or what they would look like. But I knew this child belonged to God and that eventually He would bring that child to us.

I told a few friends about this magical feeling, but it was almost too precious and too sacred to describe. I just knew that instead of this child growing in my belly, this child was growing exponentially in my heart. I felt it all so deeply that it was almost too much to bear.

Six months passed and we really began to question if we were "waiting" at the right place. *Not at all* because of the time it was taking. We just felt a tug on our hearts toward something different, so we started pursuing other options. We also started praying about using an adoption consultant. Basically an adoption middleman. Adoption consultants play a role as liaison between the family and adoption agencies. By going this route, we would not work with just one person who would walk us through everything. We would be able to connect with up to fifteen agencies at one time.

Ironically, about the same time, my sister Mary was feeling the same way we were. I called her one afternoon to spill the beans and she just sighed. I wasn't sure if the sigh was disappointment because she thought I was giving up or something else. Then she said, "I'm so glad, because I've been feeling the same thing and I wasn't sure how to tell you."

Say what?

So together, she and I made some calls. She'd used consultants in adopting Hannah, but that group had grown to be a large company and I felt more comfortable with a smaller one. It felt less commercial and more relational that way. Soon after, I found a consulting company that struck a chord with me. Mary did some research and advised me on all the questions to ask.

Through her research, we found out that one of the consultants was a good friend of my cousin Dede. After talking to Dede, who gave me the consultant's number, I made the call before I could talk myself out of it!

From the moment Genevieve answered the phone I knew, without a doubt, that God had led us to this place. Instead of being confused about why we'd felt led to stay with the other agency for six months, I trusted that it was all part of the story God was writing for us. Some of the conversations that really helped prepare us for our adoption journey had been with the agency we had signed with originally. If you find yourself at a roadblock after you've had God's peace about a big decision, just keep praying and pursuing. He'll continue to guide you. And if the road turns unexpectedly, don't waste time questioning. Just take that turn and keep pressing on.

As with any change, it meant more work had to be done. We needed to update our profile books a little, so Genevieve walked me through what needed to change and how to order more books through a different company. More copies of home studies were made, more letters were written, more paperwork was filled out, more questionnaires were answered. All of this was part of the process and worth every minute and sleepless hour it took.

We finalized everything with the adoption consulting company in October 2016. Interestingly, we mailed everything off the day before we had to evacuate for Hurricane Matthew. As Forbes was outside on a ladder working to batten down the hatches, I stood at the bottom of the ladder with our adoption paperwork, checking off comfort level questions for the consulting agency.

Unlike working with a single agency, working with a consultant means that things stay active on a daily basis. We got emails almost daily with updates and leads or situations to consider. Every week, Genevieve would find another agency she thought would be good for us based on what we were looking for. Some days, I felt weighed down by stories of children whose situations were almost unimaginable. Thankfully, we had two pediatrician friends who were willing to help us look over particular cases and give invaluable medical advice. I felt every day we were getting closer to holding the child I had loved for so long.

In November, right before Thanksgiving, we'd been emailed a case in which a mother had given birth to a baby and decided afterward it would be in the child's best interest to place her with an adoptive family. We submitted everything necessary for her to consider us as parents, including a personal email to her.

A few days later we heard that the answer was *no*. It stung a bit, but I knew that God was going to make it abundantly clear who was supposed to be ours. And this *no* was just a *no*. That's it.

The day after Thanksgiving, Genevieve called me with a special case. A child had just been born and was still in the hospital with a few medical issues. She called instead of emailing because she wanted to tell me a few things before she sent the email. One thing she wanted me to know was that he was a little Caucasian boy. I was somewhat confused, because I really couldn't shake this calling to a Hispanic child that Forbes had on his heart. But I didn't let that stop me from listening and considering this case.

The kicker for this one was that she sent a photo of him. HEARTACHE. Y'all, he was beautiful! He had tubes and wires all over him, but you could still see his chubby little cheeks. The heartache of seeing that baby laying there with no one by his side was almost too much to bear.

We received his medical records and called our pediatrician friend late that night to ask her opinion. Staying up most of the night, we prayed, talked, and considered. Was this for us or not? I couldn't imagine saying *no*, but at the same time I wanted God to make it abundantly clear that this child was for our family. If this was it, we would be taking on a medically challenged child with a lot of unknowns. This was scary to us, but we had confidence that He would equip us for whatever He required.

That night, we stayed up so late that we overslept and had a frantic morning trying to get the kids off to school. In all of the chaos, we didn't make our final decision, which we needed to do by 9 a.m.

As he headed out the door, Forbes turned. "I'm going to call you when I get to the office," he promised.

When he left to drop the kids off at school, I dropped to the floor and prayed and prayed that God would guide Forbes. He was the spiritual leader of our home and whatever God placed on his heart, I trusted.

That said, leaving the decision in God's hands was pretty hard for me. Every time I closed my eyes, that squishy little face kept showing up.

After a long conversation on the phone with Forbes and talking out many things, he felt strongly that this situation was not for us. There were many reasons, and I knew that much prayer had gone into his decision. So although hearing *no* was hard, it was right.

I hung up the phone. I thanked God for direction and for the wisdom he had given Forbes. Then, I cried.

After pulling myself together, I called Genevieve to let her know that we were not 100 percent sure why, but this child was not for us. For hours after that decision, I had a yucky feeling. I knew we'd made the right choice, but I couldn't get that baby's face out of my mind. I spent several hours alone, needing quiet time with God. Then, when I was ready to talk, I called my sister Mary to update her.

Mary knew me well enough to leave me be until I was ready to share. We chatted for a few minutes before I told her how I felt. Then we sat there and both made lunch together while still on the phone. For some reason we were both eating egg salad that day, which we found kind of funny. As we were talking, I got a call on the other line. I told her someone from Louisiana was calling me and that I'd call her back in a minute.

When I clicked over to say *hello*, the person on the other line spoke first.

"Sarah?"

"Yes, ma'am. This is Sarah."

The sound on the phone was odd. It sounded almost like a telemarketer. But it wasn't a telemarketer. I was on speaker phone with five women.

The woman who spoke early did so again. "Hi," she said, "this is Teresa from a private adoption agency, and we have a situation here we'd like to tell you about."

My whole body went warm. Chills rolled down my spine. My feet went out from under me.

I plopped down on the bench in our foyer and listened as she said they had a birth mother whom we matched with. I couldn't believe what I was hearing as I tried to focus to catch every detail. She told me they had a dear client they'd grown quite fond of who was expecting a biracial, Hispanic baby girl due in four weeks. Teresa went over all the information about the case and then mentioned the birth mother probably wouldn't go all four weeks. I tried to take in the fact that I was about to have a baby girl in a month or less. We talked for a few more minutes and then hung up. I was in disbelief that this very morning we painfully but obediently said *no* to something for reasons we didn't quite understand. Four hours later we had a MATCH!

{ *chapter thirteen* }

IN OUR ARMS

A child born to another woman calls me Mom.
The depth of that tragedy and the magnitude
of that privilege are not lost on me.[21]

Jody Landers

I WASN'T SURE IF I should drive to Forbes's office to tell him in person or just call him. Either way, I couldn't wait another second. So I called him and said, "Hey, can you close your door for a minute? I need to talk to you."

He said to hang on, then I heard the door close. I took a deep breath and said, "Well, what do you think about having another girl?" I began bawling over the phone.

"We matched?" he whispered.

I told him that we'd matched with a girl who was due in a month. "Babe, we are having a baby in a month!" Then, "I'm coming to your office. I just couldn't wait to tell you."

"Well," he said, "maybe you should calm down for a few before you drive."

I didn't calm down. I just laughed and hung up.

Since God is in every detail, I'll share a few details about the match process. In this particular case, the birth mother, Sadie, asked for some help from the agency in making her decision. Some birth mothers want to do it themselves, while others want help. Teresa had received our package right before Thanksgiving. After reading our profile book, she told the placement director she'd found the perfect family for Sadie's baby.

The placement director responded, "Well, there are other families who've been waiting longer and we just received this packet. Are you sure? That doesn't seem quite right."

Teresa answered, "Well, here is their profile book, you let me know what you think."

Thirty minutes later, the placement director walked into Teresa's office and asked, "How do you know these people?"

Teresa was confused. "I don't know them at all," she said. "What do you mean?"

"There is no way you don't know these people," the placement director said. "They literally said everything Sadie is looking for."

Teresa just smiled, "And now you know why I said they're a perfect match."

They gathered up two more great candidates and gave the profile books to Sadie to look over. She read through each and with tears in her eyes handed Teresa our profile book.

With finality, she said, "These are who I want."

We received our match call on Tuesday, November 29, 2016. I was supposed to leave the next day for a three-day get away with my sweet college roommate Rachel. It had been a long time since we had gotten some time together so she'd planned a little trip for us up to Asheville, North Carolina.

I couldn't decide what to do. I felt like I had so much to get done, but we'd had this trip planned for months. Forbes gently reminded me that I wouldn't be going anywhere or doing anything for quite some time once we had a newborn. He said I should just go. So, off I went.

It was a great trip. We shopped for baby stuff, and I spent hours on the phone with the agency getting information together. We also learned we needed to plan to spend Christmas in Louisiana. It wasn't looking like Sadie would make it until after Christmas and the court system might hold us up because of the holiday. My head was swimming with all sorts of information: baby names, nursery plans, celebrating Christmas in another state . . . Even with all the distractions, I'm glad Rachel and I were able to get away that weekend. My soul is always refreshed by time with my dear friend.

I rushed home that Saturday to see Audrey finish up a soccer tournament and to get her ready for her first daddy-daughter dance. Warren's plan for the evening was hot chocolate, pajamas, and a Christmas movie. My kind of guy.

Sunday evening, we sat the kids down to talk and pray with them. We prayed for their baby sister, and we talked about what things would look like when Forbes and I got the call to go get their new sibling. My little man didn't like sleeping away from home at the time, so we gave him a pep talk. The kids were going to stay with my parents while Forbes and I headed to Louisiana. That news reassured them both.

Sunday night, Forbes fell asleep on the couch around 8 p.m., which annoyed me. I had a million things to discuss with him and he just passed out. I was wired, so I started washing baby clothes. Thankfully, I'd saved all of Audrey's keepsake baby items. Around 11 p.m., I drove to my parents' house, where they were still up watching a movie. Surprised, mom asked what I was up to.

"Don't mind me," I said. "I just need a bag." I told her I couldn't sleep and that I'd washed a bunch of baby clothes, so I was going to pack our new baby's bag. Mom returned shortly with a bag, and then off I went. Before you think I'm crazy, my parents live eight houses down from us on the same street. So it was a quick outing at 11 p.m. at night! I stayed up even later that night making my "baby needs" list.

The next morning began the big shopping day when I planned to check off all the boxes. Elizabeth was going to meet me right after the kids' school drop off. Along with the usual Christmas list, we had a long list of baby items and a local ministry to buy for. It was a MEGA shopping list. We knew the baby could come in the next few weeks, so we had decided Monday was the day to get everything done. We planned to shop our way through every store from Sam's to Target. If we timed it right, we would even have time for coffee and a quick lunch before time to pick the kids up from school.

I went to bed much later than normal, hoping I hadn't forgotten anything. At 4:30 a.m., I was woken abruptly by Forbes. I've never seen his eyes so big in my life. He leaned over and said, "She's in labor." I'd been in a dead sleep, so it took me about thirty seconds to comprehend what he was talking about. Then we both jumped up.

The next few minutes played out like a scene from a movie. We both paced the length of the bed before meeting each other in the middle to hug excitedly and ask, "What do we do now?" We hadn't gotten this far in our plan.

Forbes ran to his office to get on the phone with Delta about flights. While we knew where the agency was located, we hadn't planned our trip there. It had only been five days since we were matched and we were still supposed to have a Skype session with Sadie. This was all happening so fast!

We agreed to wait until 6 a.m. before waking everyone up. In the meantime, I showered and started throwing clothes on my bed, wondering how to pack when your baby is on her way and you have no clue how long you'll be away from home. I waited until 6 a.m. on the dot and called my mom.

She answered with a question: "Do we have a baby?"

"Um, well she should be here within the next few minutes, so ... yes," I said, "almost."

Mom said she would take the kids to school and then come help me pack.

Next, I called my sister. Then I rang Elizabeth, who was asleep but guessed something was up because she knew I would never interrupt her precious sleep. Our massive shopping day had turned into *her* massive shopping day. I couldn't think straight and because my sister had experienced staying with a newborn in another state for a few weeks before, she called Elizabeth with a list of the must-haves. Together, they made a great team. Once Elizabeth got to my house after that momentous shopping trip, I had everything I needed. She helped make room for all the baby items she'd purchased at Target by rearranging the two massive suitcases I packed. Then Forbes and I were off to the airport.

On our first flight, Forbes and I finally looked at each other. It was all becoming very real. He mentioned that we hadn't even had a chance to look at any of the medical records. It had all been such a huge leap of faith, but it felt so right. We'd been praying and praying for this.

As we sat on the plane with pen and paper in hand, we

did what any expecting parents would do. We made a list of names. But we had only a few hours to make this decision, not the months you normally have. We narrowed it down to a combination of six names. When we got off the plane, we had it down to two, both of us having our own preference. We just wanted to see her face before we chose.

The hours crept by and after what felt like forever, we finally made it to the hospital. We pulled up around 8 p.m. with nothing but the baby bag I'd packed at 11 p.m. the night before. The rest of our luggage was lost by the airline, but we couldn't have cared less.

We were nervous because Sadie had asked to meet us before we saw the baby. Thankfully, our social worker had stayed at the hospital all day making sure Sadie and the baby were okay. By the time we made it there, Sadie had fallen asleep for the night. That took the edge off a little, but we were still anxious.

When we arrived to the maternity ward, they put us in a room, just as if I'd given birth. Then the wait began. We sat in that room for a good twenty minutes listening to the wheels of carts go by, each time thinking it was our baby about to come through the door. At one point, we were so sure the cart carrying our baby to us was coming down the hall that we stood up, hearts in our throats, staring at the open doorway. Then we watched as the janitor rolled by with his cart full of brooms and buckets. All we could do was laugh. It was nervous laughter, but it helped to ease a tiny bit of tension.

Finally, we heard the rolling wheels of a bassinet cart. We'd been told that no one but a nurse had held our girl so far. Before I could hold her (oh, the torture!), we had to go over a few legalities: drivers' licenses, signed paperwork, and medical bracelets that matched hers. I handed my license to the nurse and stared at the bassinet where our tiny, precious baby slept. Her mahogany complexion was beautiful. She looked like an angel, swaddled tight and wearing a cute hat, her silky black hair peeking out of the sides. The bracelet on her tiny wrist had no name, just a number.

After what seemed an agonizingly long three minutes, the moment finally came. I held our daughter for the first time at 9:28 p.m. She was not just a number anymore. She was ours. I couldn't believe this was happening. This child that God had allowed me to love for so long was finally here.

She had the perfect little face. Everything about her was beautiful: her eyes, lips, nose, and head full of hair. Now she would have a beautiful name to match. Forbes and I looked at each other and agreed that the name we'd chosen fit perfectly: *Analise Elizabeth Buck.* My mom suggested *Analise,* which means "devoted to God," and *Elizabeth* was the name of many special people in our lives. We spent the next two days getting to know our tiny little six-pound peanut.

Adoption is such a beautiful and hard thing. As I sat on a hospital bed with a sweet-smelling newborn on my chest, in another room not too far away lay a tired mother with an empty womb and empty arms. At times, it was almost too much to process. We were so grateful to spend some very special moments with Sadie at two different times while at the hospital. Both instances were hard, but I wouldn't have traded them for anything. She said the most beautiful thing when I asked if she would like to hold Analise.

She closed her eyes, then looked up at me with tears and said, "No thank you. I want to always remember her in your arms." This beautiful woman had given me a priceless treasure that cost her everything.

After those two days in the hospital, we were ready to take Analise to our new home away from home. In Louisiana, there's a three-day period during which the birth mother can change her mind about the adoption. We knew Sadie would not change her mind, but we still had one more full day to go once we left the hospital and the real approval process could begin. We heard it could be weeks before we received final approval to take our baby home, so we steeled ourselves for the wait.

Forbes found a great place for us to stay while we waited for that third day and for the days leading up to our approval to head back to our home state. On the morning of that third day, confident as we were that everything would work out, there was a heaviness. In the little studio apartment where we were staying, we signed the papers with the legal team and our amazing agency workers by our side. We sat there, without a dry eye in the room, and signed on all those dotted lines for this perfect girl to be OUR girl. We felt and acknowledged the full weight of the situation. It was not lost on me that Sadie's rights were being forever relinquished, making Analise forever not hers. It was one of the most sobering and significant moments of my life.

After that first week in Louisiana, we decided Warren and Audrey needed at least one parent to be with them, so Forbes flew home. My parents were doing an amazing job with the kids, but this would allow them to fly out and meet their granddaughter. They simply couldn't wait until we got home to meet her. After staying for a few days, they headed back, and my sister Mary came, promising to stay until we got to go home. This was incredibly generous because it meant she was missing Christmas parties, plays, and fun holiday events with her children—all to be with us.

We spent the next couple days taking Analise for her checkup at the pediatrician's office, taking her to visit the staff at the adoption agency, and fitting in a little Christmas shopping. It was the sweetest time, with my sister and Analise enjoying each other's company as we waited for the approval to go home.

After Mary had been with us a few days, we were out running a few errands with a nine-day-old when we got the long-awaited call. Actually, we missed it. But they left a message, and we listened to the voicemail at least three times in the car, cheering and crying that we were cleared to go home! It was a miracle that we got the call only nine days in. Sometimes the wait is much longer.

On December 15, Mary packed the three of us up, and we got on a plane headed home where we could all be together. Audrey and Warren finally met their new sister. What a fun day that was! It still amazes me that before we even reached Analise's due date, we were at home, all together under one roof.

As you can imagine, that year's Christmas Eve service was extra special. As I held a newborn gift from God in my arms, I remembered the hope that I'd cherished that last Christmas Eve service, which made the celebration of Jesus' birth that much richer. To think that Mary, the mother of Jesus, held the Savior of the world in her arms, and now I held this perfect promise from the One who knit her together. Beauty from ashes, indeed.

The Pelican

So, have you been wondering about the significance of the pelican was? That story is perhaps my favorite one to tell. On that first night when Mary got to Louisiana, we snuggled up on the couch with Analise to watch a Hallmark Christmas movie. Mary had the baby in her lap with her tiny feet up on her chest. I wasn't paying much attention to the movie, as the business of Analise's nursery decor was at the forefront in my mind.

Not long before all this, I'd commissioned an artist to do a painting for our home. As I sat there, I decided I wanted that same artist to do something special for Analise's new nursery. I'd fallen in love with some black-and-white baby animal prints on Etsy and that was literally all I had so far for her room. I thought I'd keep the animal theme going. Wanting to honor the place of her birth, I picked up my phone to type *Louisiana state animal* in the search. Can you even guess what appeared on the screen?

My sister glanced over at me and said, "What is wrong with you? Your face is white." I held up my phone so she could see. The very first image that came up months earlier when I looked up the symbolism of *pelican* was an image of a mama pelican with its wings expanded and three babies underneath. Well, that image is actually the Louisiana state flag. Yep. That's right, friends. The Louisiana state bird is a PELICAN!

When people wonder if God is real, stories like the pelican and Analise's adoption need to be shared. But this isn't *just* a story. This is God speaking through an intricately-crafted miracle that, in His grace, He let our family take part in. He speaks to each of us every day, but the question is, *Are we listening?* Are we taking time to pay attention to the details? None of this story

I've just told you would have made any sense if we hadn't been paying attention. We would have skipped right on over all those seemingly random events.

It's hard not to wonder after seeing Him put all of this together, what might I have missed? What other stories has He been weaving together that I didn't have the eyes to see?

Our pelican experience was a gift, because through it God reassured us that He was working and that we weren't alone in this story. Now, when things are hard or discouraging, remembering how God spoke to us then and how He graciously revealed His will to us gives us courage to push back against doubt and unbelief. We know that there will be hard moments in this journey of raising an adopted child. But the beauty and hope of walking this path is knowing God led us here. Stories like our pelican story, along with the myriad of other ways God revealed Himself to us, propel us forward without letting us get in the way.

Elaine Burge, the artist I mentioned, painted a picture for Analise's nursery. You can see how it turned out on the front of this book. That beautiful painting hung over her crib when she was a baby, and it still hangs in her room now. It is a daily reminder to our family that God writes beautiful stories. He is the master storyteller. We just have to keep our eyes open to see His tales unfold.

I still look back and marvel at how God graciously led us through a wilderness long before the pelicans and the path to Analise. Through my illness, He taught our family what it looks like to wait for Him even when things are painful and confusing. And we know now that when we can't see how He's going to get us out of the mess we're in, all the while He's making things beautiful. But in *His* time, not ours.

I see now that those long months of illness enabled me to fully participate in the richness and fullness of God bringing Analise into our lives. We are not the same people we were when we first started this journey. God has shaped us through the mystery and uncertainty of that incredibly hard season, ultimately making us wiser and more free. I truly believe I had to experience the suffering and losses from Lyme in order to appreciate the depth and beauty of Analise's adoption.

Friend, my hope for you is that, years from now, you too will be able to look back and say with joy, "I see it now!"[22] Be patient, because He who began a good work in you will be faithful to complete it (Philippians 1:6). And when all the broken pieces of the mosaic of your life begin to come together and you realize He's been at work framing His masterpiece all along, my prayer is that *you will see what I've seen:*

That He is undeniably real and infinitely good.

GRATITUDE

All my words fall short
I got nothing new
How could I express
All my gratitude?
I could sing these songs
As I often do
But every song must end
And You never do
So I throw up my hands
And praise You again and again
'Cause all that I have is a hallelujah
Hallelujah
And I know it's not much
But I've nothing else fit for a King
Except for a heart singing hallelujah
Hallelujah
I've got one response
I've got just one move
With my arm stretched wide
I will worship You
So I throw up my hands
And praise You again and again
'Cause all that I have is a hallelujah
Hallelujah
And I know it's not much
But I've nothing else fit for a King
Except for a heart singing hallelujah
Hallelujah

-Brandon Lake

THANK YOU

Thank you, Lord, for this beautiful,
messy story that you gave us.
Thank You for your unending love, grace, and mercy.
Thank You for loving me despite my *I-got-this* mentality.
The truth is I have nothing and am nothing without You.

*There is absolutely no way to put into words my sincerest gratitude
to all of those God placed on this journey with us.*

Thank you . . .

To my faithful prayer warriors, then and now, who had the words to pray when we did not. To those who fasted, pleaded, knitted, wept, cooked, visited, and kept the text messages going. To those who made special arrangements and called in favors to friends and doctors. To all the doctors that we met along the way, for the efforts you made to find answers. To those of you who silently, graciously carried our burdens. To those who offered sound, bold advice when it was hard to hear. To those who never left our side, when it would have been so much easier to leave. To those who drove, watched, loved on, or played with our kids.

To those who joyfully and obediently joined our adoption story. For all the phone calls, the calls made on our behalf, the advice, the prayers, the encouragement, the research, and the hope. For all of you who loved us well then and continue to love us well now through whatever journey God takes us on.

And lastly, to those who have prayed this book into fruition . . . many, many thanks. It could not have been done without your prayers and encouragement.

NOTES

1   Hillsong United. "Oceans." Zion, Hillsong Music/ Sparrow Records, 2013, track 4. Hillsong, https://hillsong. com/lyrics/oceans-where-feet-may-fail/.

2   Greear, J.D. "The Book of Ephesians by J. D. Greear, Session 9." Right Now Media, 2016, https://www.rightnow-media.org/Content/Series/195647?episode=9.

3   Stanley, Andy. Enemies of the Heart: Breaking Free from the Four Emotions That Control You. The Crown Publishing Group, 2011. Digital.

4   Chan, Francis. "The Book of James: Francis Chan." Right Now Media, 2015, https://www.rightnowmedia.org/ Content/Series/159923.

5   Warren, Rick. "Daily Hope with Rick Warren." Facebook, 21 Oct. 2015, 8:45 pm, https://www.facebook.com/ DailyHope/posts/982163598506413. Accessed November 2020.

6   Waller, John. "While I'm Waiting." The Blessing. Reunion, 2009, track 8.

7   Meyers, Joyce. "What To Do When You're Waiting On God." Joyce Meyers. Oct. 2013, http://www.joycemeyer. org/articles/ea.aspx?article=what_to_do_when_youre_waiting_on-god.

8   Lusko, Jenny. Fight to Flourish. W Publishing, 2020.

9   Whitaker, Nicole. "The Answer to End All Questions." GirlTalk. 9 Sept. 2013, http://girltalkhome.com/blog/ the-answer-to-end-all-questions/.

10 Driscoll, Mark. *Who Do You Think You Are?* Thomas Nelson, Inc., 2013.

11 "Under Our Skin." Dir. Andy Abrahams Wilson. Am-

azon Prime Web, 2009. 20 November 2014.

12 Casey, Lara. *Cultivate*. Thomas Nelson, 2017.

13 John F. Conner, Lemarchand, R [Rosalynde]. Inspirational Poetry [pinterest post]. October 2020, https://i.pinimg.com/originals/9b/99/06/9b9906a2949d-9d966756c1698342487a.jpg

14 Lewis, C.S. The Problem of Pain. Harper One, 2001.

15 Lusko, Levi, pastor. "Not Quickly Broken: Becoming Antifragile." Fresh Life Church, iTunes app, 27 January 2020.

16 Furtick, Steven, pastor. "Ghosted." Elevation with Steven Furtick, iTunes app, 27 January 2020.

17 Daniels, Dharius, guest speaker. "I See It Now." Elevation with Steven Furtick, iTunes app, 1 November 2020.

18 Furtick, Steven, pastor. "Ghosted." Elevation with Steven Furtick, iTunes app, 27 January 2020.

19 Vanauken, Sheldon, Severe Mercy. Harper One, 1987.

20 "Pelicans." Wikipedia, Wikipedia Foundation, October 2015, https://en.wikipedia.org/wiki/Pelican.

21 Landers, Jody. "Thoughtful Thursday: Adoption." The Lettered Cottage. 18 November 2015, https://theletteredcottage.net/thought-full-thursday-adoption/.

22 Daniels, Dharius, guest speaker. "I See It Now." Elevation with Steven Furtick, iTunes app, 1 November 2020.

CPSIA information can be obtained
at www.ICGtesting.com
Printed in the USA
FSHW011941210421
80714FS